The Legacy and Impact of Podiatric Fellowship Training

Editors

THOMAS ZGONIS
CHRISTOPHER F. HYER

CLINICS IN PODIATRIC MEDICINE AND SURGERY

www.podiatric.theclinics.com

Consulting Editor
THOMAS J. CHANG

April 2022 • Volume 39 • Number 2

ELSEVIER

1600 John F. Kennedy Boulevard • Suite 1800 • Philadelphia, Pennsylvania, 19103-2899

http://www.theclinics.com

CLINICS IN PODIATRIC MEDICINE AND SURGERY Volume 39, Number 2
April 2022 ISSN 0891-8422, ISBN-13: 978-0-323-84963-0

Editor: Lauren Boyle
Developmental Editor: Diana Grace Ang

Clinics in Podiatric Medicine and Surgery (ISSN 0891-8422) is published quarterly by Elsevier Inc., 360 Park Avenue South, New York, NY 10010-1710. Months of issue are January, April, July, and October. Business and Editorial Offices: 1600 John F. Kennedy Blvd., Ste. 1800, Philadelphia, PA 19103-2899. Customer Service Office: 3251 Riverport Lane, Maryland Heights, MO 63043. Periodicals postage paid at New York, NY and additional mailing offices. Subscription prices are $319.00 per year for US individuals, $773.00 per year for US institutions, $100.00 per year for US students and residents, $393.00 per year for Canadian individuals, $796.00 for Canadian institutions, $476.00 for international individuals, $796.00 per year for international institutions, $100.00 per year for Canadian students/residents, and $220.00 per year for foreign students/residents. To receive student/resident rate, orders must be accompanied by name of affiliated institution, date of term, and the *signature* of program/residency coordinator on institution letterhead. Orders will be billed at individual rate until proof of status is received. Foreign air speed delivery is included in all *Clinics* subscription prices. All prices are subject to change without notice. POSTMASTER: Send address changes to *Clinics in Podiatric Medicine and Surgery*, Elsevier Health Sciences Division, Subscription Customer Service, 3251 Riverport Lane, Maryland Heights, MO 63043. **Customer Service: 1-800-654-2452 (US). From outside of the US, call 314-447-8871. Fax: 314-447-8029. E-mail: JournalsCustomerService-usa@elsevier.com (for print support); JournalsOnlineSupport-usa@elsevier.com (for online support).**

Reprints. For copies of 100 or more of articles in this publication, please contact the Commercial Reprints Department, Elsevier Inc., 360 Park Avenue South, New York, NY 10010-1710. Tel.: 212-633-3874; Fax: 212-633-3820; E-mail: reprints@elsevier.com.

Clinics in Podiatric Medicine and Surgery is covered in *MEDLINE/PubMed (Index Medicus)* and *EMBASE/Excerpta Medica*.

Contributors

CONSULTING EDITOR

THOMAS J. CHANG, DPM
Clinical Professor and Past Chairman, Department of Podiatric Surgery, California College of Podiatric Medicine, Faculty, The Podiatry Institute, Redwood Orthopedic Surgery Associates, Santa Rosa, California, USA

EDITORS

THOMAS ZGONIS, DPM, FACFAS
Professor and Director, Reconstructive Foot and Ankle Surgery Fellowship, Division of Podiatric Medicine and Surgery, Department of Orthopaedics, University of Texas Health San Antonio, Joe R. & Teresa Lozano Long School of Medicine, San Antonio, Texas, USA

CHRISTOPHER F. HYER, DPM, MS, FACFAS
Fellowship Trained Foot and Ankle Surgeon, Board Certified, Foot and Ankle Reconstructive Surgery, Fellowship Co-Director, Advanced Foot and Ankle Reconstruction, Orthopedic Foot and Ankle Center, Fellow, American College of Foot and Ankle Surgeons, Past Board of Directors, American College of Foot and Ankle Surgeons, Foot and Ankle Surgery, Masters Science, Clinical Research, Drexel School of Medicine, Worthington, Ohio, USA; Fellowship Director, Orthopedic Foot and Ankle Center, Columbus, Ohio, USA

AUTHORS

ROBERTO BRANDÃO, DPM, AACFAS
The Centers for Advanced Orthopaedics, Orthopaedic Associates of Central Maryland Division, Catonsville, Maryland, USA

HANI M. BADAHDAH, DPM, MD, MS
Consultant Podiatric Foot and Ankle Surgery, Dr. Edrees Specialized Medical Center, Jeddah, Saudi Arabia; Diabetes and Endocrinology Center, King Fahd Specialist Hospital, Buraydah, Saudi Arabia

RONALD BELCZYK, DPM
Foot and Ankle Specialist, Center for Foot Surgery, Oxnard, Oxnard, California, USA

BRAD BUSSEWITZ, DPM, FACFAS
Fellowship Trained Foot and Ankle Surgeon, Board Certified, Foot andAnkle Reconstructive Surgery, Steindler Orthopedic Clinic, Iowa City, Iowa, USA

DEVON CONSUL, DPM, BSN, AACFAS
Fellow, Orthopedic Foot and Ankle Center, Worthington, Ohio, USA

JAMES M. COTTOM, DPM, FACFAS
Fellowship Trained Foot and Ankle Surgeon, Fellowship Director, Florida Orthopedic Foot and Ankle Center, Sarasota, Florida, USA

WILLIAM T. DECARBO, DPM, FACFAS
Fellowship Trained Foot and Ankle Surgeon, Board Certified, Foot and Ankle
Reconstructive Surgery, St. Clair Orthopedic Associates, Pittsburgh, Pennsylvania,
USA

JASON GEORGE DEVRIES, DPM, FACFAS
Fellowship Trained Foot and Ankle Surgeon, Board Certified, Foot and Ankle
Reconstructive Surgery, Orthopedics and Sports Medicine BayCare Clinic, Manitowoc,
Wisconsin, USA

MICHAEL D. DUJELA, DPM, FACFAS
Fellowship Trained Foot and Ankle Surgeon, Board Certified, Foot and Ankle
Reconstructive Surgery, Fellowship Director, Advanced Foot and Ankle Surgical
Fellowship, Washington Orthopaedic Center, Centralia, Washington, USA

COREY M. FIDLER, DPM, AACFAS
Fellowship Trained Foot and Ankle Surgeon, Assistant Professor, Department of
Orthopaedic Surgery, Virginia Tech Carilion School of Medicine, Roanoke, Virginia,
USA

CHRISTOPHER F. HYER, DPM, MS, FACFAS
Fellowship Trained Foot and Ankle Surgeon, Board Certified, Foot and Ankle
Reconstructive Surgery, Fellowship Co-Director, Advanced Foot and Ankle
Reconstruction, Orthopedic Foot and Ankle Center, Fellow, American College of Foot and
Ankle Surgeons, Past Board of Directors, American College of Foot and Ankle Surgeons,
Foot and Ankle Surgery, Masters Science, Clinical Research, Drexel School of Medicine,
Worthington, Ohio, USA; Fellowship Director, Orthopedic Foot and Ankle Center,
Columbus, Ohio, USA

TRAVIS LANGAN, DPM, AACFAS
Fellowship Trained Foot and Ankle Surgeon, Board Certified, Foot and Ankle
Reconstructive Surgery, Carle Orthopedics and Sports Medicine, Champaign, Illinois,
USA

JEFFREY E. MCALISTER, DPM, FACFAS
Fellowship Trained Foot and Ankle Surgeon, Phoenix Foot and Ankle Institute, Scottsdale,
Arizona, USA

SHRUNJAY R. PATEL, DPM, AACFAS
Assistant Professor, Division of Vascular Surgery, Department of Surgery, The University
of North Carolina at Chapel Hill, Chapel Hill, North Carolina, USA

MARK A. PRISSEL, DPM, FACFAS
Fellowship Trained Foot and Ankle Surgeon, Board Certified, Foot and Ankle
Reconstructive Surgery, Fellowship Director, Orthopedic Foot and Ankle Center,
Columbus, Ohio, USA; Orthopedic Foot and Ankle Center, Worthington, Ohio, USA

CRYSTAL L. RAMANUJAM, DPM, MSc, FACFAS
Associate Professor/Clinical, Division of Podiatric Medicine and Surgery, Department of
Orthopaedics, University of Texas Health San Antonio, San Antonio, Texas, USA

RYAN T. SCOTT, DPM, FACFAS
Fellowship Trained Foot and Ankle Surgeon, Board Certified, Foot and Ankle
Reconstructive Surgery, Fellowship Director, The CORE Institute Foot and Ankle
Reconstruction Fellowship, The CORE Institute, Phoenix, Arizona, USA

KIMIA SOHRABI, DPM
Foot and Ankle Specialist, Foot and Ankle Centers of North Houston, Houston, Texas, USA

MATTHEW D. SORENSEN, DPM, FACFAS
Weil Foot & Ankle Institute, Libertyville, Illinois, USA

JOHN J. STAPLETON, DPM, FACFAS
Chief, Division of Podiatric Surgery, LVPG Orthopedics and Sports Medicine, Lehigh Valley Health Network, Allentown, Pennsylvania, USA; Clinical Assistant Professor of Surgery, Penn State College of Medicine, Hershey, Pennsylvania, USA

ALAN C. STUTO, DPM, FACFAS
LVPG Orthopedics and Sports Medicine, Lehigh Valley Health Network, Bethlehem, Pennsylvania, USA

STEVEN L. STUTO, DPM
Adjunct Faculty and Fellow in Reconstructive Foot and Ankle Surgery, Division of Podiatric Medicine and Surgery, Department of Orthopaedics, University of Texas Health San Antonio, San Antonio, Texas, USA

MITCHELL THOMPSON, DPM, AACFAS
Fellow, Orthopedic Foot and Ankle Center, Worthington, Ohio, USA

BRYAN VAN DYKE, DO
Orthopedic Surgeon, Fellowship Trained Foot and Ankle Surgeon, Summit Orthopaedics, Idaho Falls, Idaho, USA

THOMAS ZGONIS, DPM, FACFAS
Professor and Director, Reconstructive Foot and Ankle Surgery Fellowship, Division of Podiatric Medicine and Surgery, Department of Orthopaedics, University of Texas Health San Antonio, Joe R. and Teresa Lozano Long School of Medicine, San Antonio, Texas, USA

Contents

> Fusion of the first metatarsophalangeal joint has been used by foot and
> ankle surgeons as a reproducible and useful means of treating end-
> stage arthritis of the great toe. However, the overall utility and successful
> outcomes of this procedure have led to its incorporation into the treatment
> of more significant bunion deformities, reconstruction forefoot, and
> salvage procedures. The authors review surgical fixation methods, offer
> insightful technical pearls for challenging cases and share examples of
> complex reconstructive and salvage procedures.

> Lesser toe plantar plate injuries at the metatarsophalangeal (MTP) joint are a
> common source of metatarsalgia. Chronic pain with weight-bearing is the
> common presentation of lesser toe instability. Deformity occurs when the
> plantar plate is torn or attenuated. Crossover toe and MTP instability often
> occur with multiplane deformity, most commonly with dorsal contracture
> of the second toe and medial drift over the Hallux. In this article, the authors
> present a comprehensive stepwise approach to diagnosing and treating
> plantar plate injuries using both dorsal and plantar approach techniques.

> There has been significant enhancement in surgical management of hallux
> valgus deformity. Recognition of the role of medial column hypermobility
> has resulted in better functional outcomes with decreased risk of recur-
> rence. Modern techniques have evolved to include enhanced fixation in a
> move toward minimal postoperative downtime. Evolution to include true
> triplane correction, including frontal plane derotation of the first ray, has re-
> sulted in optimal functional outcomes. The addition of anatomic triplane
> restoration, enhanced internal fixation, and early return to weight-bearing
> activities are combined resulting in lifelong correction with excellent func-
> tional outcomes and a high degree of patient satisfaction.

effective multidisciplinary team for the treatment of the diabetic foot analogous to that seen in elite team sports.

The concept of surgical offloading with external fixation is especially relevant when managing diabetic patients with lower extremity wounds refractory to conservative treatment with traditional offloading. This article provides a case report and review of external fixation as a powerful device in accelerating wound healing and providing correction of osseous deformities simultaneously in the diabetic foot.

CLINICS IN PODIATRIC MEDICINE AND SURGERY

SERIES OF RELATED INTEREST

Orthopedic Clinics
https://www.orthopedic.theclinics.com/
Clinics in Sports Medicine
https://www.sportsmed.theclinics.com/
Foot and Ankle Clinics
https://www.foot.theclinics.com/
Physical Medicine and Rehabilitation Clinics
https://www.pmr.theclinics.com/

THE CLINICS ARE AVAILABLE ONLINE!
Access your subscription at:
www.theclinics.com

Foreword

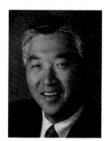

Thomas J. Chang, DPM
Consulting Editor

When I first graduated from residency training in 1993, my residency partner was fortunate to do an AO fellowship with Dr Ted Hansen. The surgical fellowships at that time were mainly linked to the AO organization, and many of them existed outside the United States. They varied from 6 weeks to 6 months.

Formal Fellowship Training in Podiatry first started in 2008. This training involves areas of Reconstructive Foot and Ankle Surgery, Limb Deformity Correction, Trauma, Diabetic Care and Reconstruction, Sports Medicine, Biomechanics, and Orthoplastics. This extra year of specialized training offers considerable exposure to advanced techniques and skills, not always covered in many residency training programs.

At the time of this publication, there are 67 fellowships either "recognized" through either the American College of Foot and Ankle Surgeons (ACFAS) or "accredited" through the Council of Podiatric Medical Education (CPME). For accreditation through the CPME, the fellowship is required to have an affiliation with a hospital or academic health center. Many of these exist within the Podiatric Medical Colleges and major University Health Care Centers.

A recent article published in the *Journal of Foot and Ankle Surgery* in 2021[1], during the 6-year period of 2013 to 2019, reported that 279 articles from Fellowship programs were published in peer-reviewed journals. That is almost 50 articles each year. Research and publication in peer-reviewed literature continues to be one requirement in many of the programs. That is one of the requirements of the ACFAS recognized programs. One-third of graduating fellows also publish again within the first 5 to 10 years of practice.

There are likely an additional 20 or more programs that are not accredited or recognized with either organization, yet still exist with the promise of providing additional training and experience to willing recipients. The quality of these training programs is not closely regulated or possible to evaluate. It is hopeful these programs will all become accredited or recognized in the future and that all Fellows can be assured their program will provide an exceptional level of training.

Clin Podiatr Med Surg 39 (2022) xiii–xiv
https://doi.org/10.1016/j.cpm.2022.03.001
0891-8422/22/© 2022 Published by Elsevier Inc.

podiatric.theclinics.com

I commend Drs Hyer and Zgonis for creating this issue with significant contributions from many current fellows in high-quality programs. These topics showcase the tremendous level of training and education many programs offer today. I hope you enjoy this issue and share an excitement to the level of Fellowship training available to our residents.

Thomas J. Chang, DPM
Redwood Orthopedic Surgery Associates
208 Concourse Boulevard
Santa Rosa, CA 95403, USA

E-mail address:
thomaschang14@comcast.net

REFERENCES

1. Casciato DJ, Thompson J, Hyer CF. Postfellowship foot and ankle surgeon research productivity: a systematic review. J Foot Ankle Surg 2022. https://doi.org/10.1053/j.jfas.2021.12.028.

Preface

The Legacy and Impact of Podiatric Fellowship Training

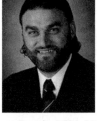

Thomas Zgonis, DPM, FACFAS   Christopher F. Hyer, DPM, MS, FACFAS
Editors

Advanced fellowship training is well recognized in allopathic/osteopathic medicine and surgery programs where trainees hone expertise and skills to further expand and focus on their chosen specialty. This is when general surgeons concentrate to become specialists, such as vascular surgeons, general orthopedists focusing on spine surgery, and likewise, broad medical disciplines, such as an internist becoming a rheumatologist.

Podiatric fellowships provide subspecialty training to individuals seeking additional surgical and/or research experience beyond residency, and with several programs now available across the country, highly qualified applicants can choose specific training that matches their career goals. The emergence of true, year-long specialized fellowship training in the podiatric surgery arena started about 25 years ago, with significant growth and demand seen over the last 5 to 10 years. Many of these fellowships offer high-volume focused training in various specialty areas, such as total ankle arthroplasty, lower-extremity trauma, complex deformity correction, diabetic limb salvage and advanced soft tissue management techniques, elite-level sports medicine, and scholarly research.

Fellowship directors bestow a unique perspective, as they are most often the experts in their field; therefore, the instruction they provide in surgery and research is invaluable. Fellowship mentorship extends far beyond didactics and surgical skills, often in the form of important daily life lessons and experiences. Fellows are getting the opportunity to meet other experts in their field and networking through national and international travel to conferences for research presentations. Continuous interaction within different specialties, such as orthopedics, plastic surgery, internal medicine, cardiology, nephrology, infectious disease, emergency room physicians, and many others, provides the fellow an irreplaceable experience and confidence that will enhance their future practice.

Clin Podiatr Med Surg 39 (2022) xv–xvi
https://doi.org/10.1016/j.cpm.2022.01.001
0891-8422/22/© 2022 Published by Elsevier Inc.

podiatric.theclinics.com

In the setting of a residency training program, the fellow is also complementing and assisting with the resident training through academics, surgery, clinical work, and research. The self-motivation of the fellow to obtain as much instruction as possible in a limited amount of time also motivates the fellowship director to stay up-to-date and teach more to all trainees involved within the program, including international fellows, residents, and students in an exciting learning environment. While the training and hours are rigorous and long, the experience gained is both unparalleled and unforgettable.

In this *Clinics in Podiatric Medicine and Surgery* issue, Dr Hyer and I are excited to collaborate with many of our past fellows to highlight various topics in reconstructive foot and ankle surgery and diabetic limb salvage disciplines. We are both fortunate to be actively involved in two of the longest running, multidisciplinary fellowships in podiatric foot and ankle surgery. We are also honored and humbled to continue to work with supremely dedicated fellows each and every year, all of whom continue to take the training and experience to another level to not only help patients but also strengthen our profession and train others.

Thomas Zgonis, DPM, FACFAS
Division of Podiatric Medicine and Surgery
Department of Orthopaedics
University of Texas Health
San Antonio Long School of Medicine
San Antonio, TX 78229, USA

Christopher F. Hyer, DPM, MS, FACFAS
Advanced Foot and Ankle Reconstruction
Orthopedic Foot and Ankle Center
Worthington, OH 43085, USA

E-mail addresses:
zgonis@uthscsa.edu (T. Zgonis)
hyerofac@gmail.com (C.F. Hyer)

High Utility of the 1st Metatarsal Phalangeal Joint Fusion

Mark A. Prissel, DPM, FACFAS[a],*, Roberto Brandão, DPM, AACFAS[b],
Michael D. Dujela, DPM, FACFAS[c], Corey M. Fidler, DPM, AACFAS[d],
Travis Langan, DPM, AACFAS[e], Christopher F. Hyer, DPM, MS, FACFAS[a]

KEYWORDS

- Bunion • Foot arthritis • Great toe pain • Foot fusion • 1st MTP arthritis • Bone graft
- Big toe arthritis

KEY POINTS

- Fusion of the first metatarsophalangeal joint can be an effective and definitive solution to painful arthritis, deformity, and salvage procedure of the great toe
- Supplemental bone graft, including from the calcaneus, can aid in defect filling, and help with fusion healing
- Various hardware can be used to achieve successful fusion including screws, plates, and compressive staples
- Overall long-term outcomes demonstrate high fusion and satisfaction rates
- Structural allograft or autograft may be necessary in revision cases with residual defects

INTRODUCTION

Arthrodesis of the first metatarsal phalangeal joint (MTP) has been used to treat end-stage hallux rigidus, hallux varus, severe hallux valgus deformities, inflammatory, and revisions for failed arthroplasties.[1–3] Initially described in the late 1800s as a successful means of treatment of hallux rigidus, foot, and ankle surgeons now use the procedure to treat a broader list of forefoot pathologies.[4] The high utility of the procedure can be attributed to its overall successful outcomes and fusion rates reported around 88% to 100%.[5–7] Various fixation methods and hardware have been described to achieve this optimal fusion rate including screw, dorsal locking plates, and staple fixation. The

[a] Orthopedic Foot and Ankle Center, 350 W Wilson Bridge Road, Suite 200, Worthington, OH 43085, USA; [b] The Centers for Advanced Orthopaedics, Orthopaedic Associates of Central Maryland Division, 910 Frederick Road, Catonsville, MD 21228, USA; [c] Washington Orthopaedic Center, 1900 Cooks Hill Road, Centralia, WA 98512, USA; [d] Department of Orthopaedic Surgery, Virginia Tech Carilion School of Medicine, 3 Riverside Circle, Roanoke, VA 24016, USA; [e] Carle Orthopaedics and Sports Medicine, 2300 South 1st Street, Champaign, IL 61820, USA
* Corresponding author.
E-mail address: markprissel@gmail.com

Clin Podiatr Med Surg 39 (2022) 157–165
https://doi.org/10.1016/j.cpm.2021.11.002
0891-8422/22/© 2021 Elsevier Inc. All rights reserved.

authors review the various application and fixation methods used by foot and surgeons for 1st MTP arthrodesis. The primary benefit of fusion is the resolution of pain, increased stability of the entire medial column, and enhanced gait.[8] Refinement of optimal fusion alignment and fixation over the time has resulted in a dependable, reproducible procedure with high patient satisfaction.[1]

HALLUX RIGIDUS

Arthritis of the 1st MTP is a common and longstanding painful pathology of the first ray often requiring the intervention of various forms. End-stage arthritis of the 1st MTP has done well with surgical arthrodesis.[5–7] For patients with longstanding pain, limited range of motion throughout the joint, and of advancing age, fusion of the joint can provide a definitive solution that reduces pain. Different methods of fixation have been used including crossed screws, dorsal locking plates, and staple fixation. Traditionally, lag screw and Steinmann pins were used as forms of fixation but lower union rates lead to a transition of dorsal locking plates with and without lag cross-screw fixation. Dorsal plating has become one of the most preferred constructs for foot and ankle surgeons performing 1st MTP arthrodesis due to its high fusion rates and allowance of immediate weight bearing.[7,9–11] Recently, staple fixation has become a popular method fixation for 1st MTP arthrodesis as it allows for less dissection and possible quicker operating times with equally satisfying fusion rates. Choudhary and colleagues found excellent fusion rates (96.7%) and outcomes in patients undergoing 1st MTP arthrodesis with 2 compression staples. Only one nonunion was reported in the study.[12]

It is crucial to consider the patient's goals in surgical decision making for hallux rigidus deformity. In some instances, a patient with moderate to significant arthritis may be a good candidate for an attempt at joint preservation via cheilectomy. The discussion should involve the probability of the progression of the disease and potential for additional surgery in the future. While many patients expect complete pain relief and restoration of motion after cheilectomy or other joint preservation techniques, this is often unrealistic. If the patient is not tolerant of the potential for revision or additional procedures, first MTP fusion should be considered the primary surgical procedure of choice.

Incisional placement directly dorsal or dorsomedial to the 1st MTPJ allows for adequate exposure of the joint. Care is taken to protect the extensor hallucis longus and brevis tendon. The joint capsule is incised to expose the 1st metatarsal head and base of the proximal phalanx. Any osteophytes are removed with a saw or rongeur. Any joint adhesions are released and the sesamoid apparatus can be released. Be sure to leave the attachment of the adductor hallucis muscle on the lateral side of the proximal phalanx when possible. After the arthrodesis procedure, this muscle will create a corrective pull of the 1st ray to help reduce the intermetatarsal angle.[13] The cartilage can be resected with joint curettage, or by using cup and cone reamers. Once the cartilage is removed, the subchondral plate is penetrated with a solid core drill and fish-scaled with an osteotome. Care is taken to preserve 1st ray length. The hallux is reduced on the metatarsal and temporary fixation can allow for the surgeon to check the reduction in all planes. A footplate can be used to check the sagittal plane. The toe should sit lightly on the footplate when the forefoot is loaded. In certain cases, a slight amount of dorsiflexion may be preferable.

Currently, for staples fixation, surgeons can use 2 compression-type staples oriented at 90° from each other across the fusion site. Additionally, a hybrid technique can be used with a lag screw and dorsal compression staples. After temporary fixation is achieved and assessed, 2 staples can be inserted after predrilled on the dorsal and medial aspect of the joint. Additionally, the temporary fixation wire can be used as a cannulated insertional technique for a traditional lag screw with supplemental dorsal staple fixation as shown in **Fig. 3**. In this setting, the staples are oriented from the dorsomedial and dorsolateral aspect of the joint with slight convergence approximately 60° from each other (**Fig. 1**).

For plate fixation, please see the hallux valgus section for images and technique.

HALLUX VALGUS

Hallux valgus remains a very common diagnosis that requires surgical treatment. Arthrodesis of the 1st metatarsophalangeal joint remains a viable and well-documented procedure for both primary and revision hallux valgus cases.[13–18] In the hallux valgus treatment workup, surgeons must consider many things in selecting the correct surgical treatment. Arthrodesis of the 1st MTPJ can correct a hallux valgus deformity and address joint pain in one procedure. It has been shown that an arthrodesis procedure can correct large intermetatarsal angle and hallux abductus angle deformities with great success.[13–18] In patients with first ray insufficiency, shortened first ray, and lesser metatarsalgia pain, arthrodesis of the first MTPJ can create stability of the medial foot and provide pain relief.[8,19]

Technique

Incisional placement directly dorsal or dorsomedial to the 1st MTPJ allows for adequate exposure of the joint. The joint is prepared in a similar fashion, denuding all cartilage surfaces and contouring all osteophytes to aid in appropriate placement of fixation. Care is taken, especially in valgus cases, to appreciate the varying degree

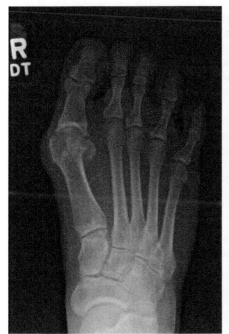
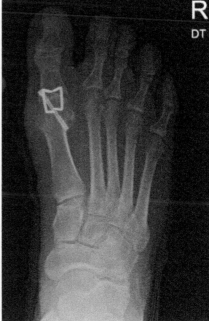

Fig. 1. 63-year-old female with a hallux valgus and rigidus deformity treated with arthrodesis using a cross-compression screw and 2 dorsal staples for fixation.

of bony integrity at different aspects of the MTP joint. In these cases, the medial aspect of the metatarsal head is relatively soft as deformity does not significantly load the medial side of the joint relative to the lateral side. Typically the bone at the proximal phalanx base is much harder than the bone on the side of the metatarsal head. Over-zealous joint preparation, either with reamers or hand instrumentation, can result in substantial bone loss requiring intercalary grafting. Be sure to leave the attachment of the adductor hallucis muscle on the lateral side of the proximal phalanx. Oftentimes, however, a distal soft tissue procedure may be required to appropriately reduce the deformities in the transverse and coronal planes. Although the adductor hallucis is maintained, the release of the fibular suspensory ligament can be performed, as well as, fenestration of the lateral 1st MTP capsule. After the arthrodesis procedure, this muscle will create a corrective pull of the 1st ray to help reduce the intermetatarsal angle.[13] Care is taken to preserve 1st ray length. The hallux is reduced on the metatarsal and temporary fixation can allow for the surgeon to check the reduction in all planes. A footplate can be used to check the sagittal plane. The toe should sit lightly on the footplate when the forefoot is loaded. In certain cases, a slight amount of dorsiflexion may be preferable. Once adequate reduction is achieved, fixation of choice can be performed. Fixation options range from cross-screws, staples, plate, and to any combination of the above. **Figs. 2** and **3** show adequate reduction and correction of a severe bunion deformity. Note the hallux is aligned in the sagittal plane as well to allow for toe purchase (see **Figs. 2** and **3**).

FAILED IMPLANTS AND REVISIONS

The use of 1st MTP implants is widely accepted; however, failed implants can create a problem for many patients. 1st MTP arthrodesis is an important tool for salvage after a failed joint arthroplasty. The use of bulk allograft or autograft can be useful to fill bone voids left after a failed implant. 1st MTP arthrodesis has been shown to be very successful in implant failure cases.[20–22] There are many products available for allograft options and they range from small bone plugs to replace synthetic cartilage grafts to large bulk cylindrical grafts. Autograft can also be an option. Tricortical structural graft can be obtained from the calcaneus or iliac crest. Preoperative evaluation, weight-bearing radiographs, and advanced imaging should be used to develop an operative plan before the procedure.

Additionally, 1st MTP fusion is an appropriate consideration for failed hallux valgus correction or failed cheilectomy, even when the appropriate bone stock remains. Moreover, when severe lesser toe and lesser metatarsal deformity is present or failed lesser ray surgery a 1st MTP fusion may be coupled with a lesser metatarsal head resection of 2 to 5 and hammertoe corrective procedures. This approach may be considered for revision surgery even in patients with nonrheumatoid (**Fig. 4**).

Technique

The joint is accessed in the same fashion. Removal of the implant will leave a variable-sized void. The appropriate graft should allow for adequate length and alignment of

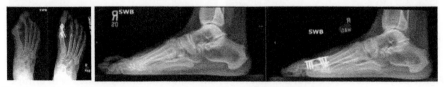

Fig. 2. Severe bunion deformity corrected using 1st MPJ arthrodesis.

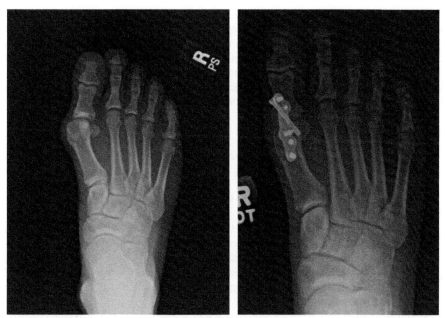

Fig. 3. A patient with painful range of motion and hallux valgus deformity of the 1st MTP treated with arthrodesis. Calcaneal bone graft was used to enhance healing. The patient was back to presurgical activity at 3-months postoperative.

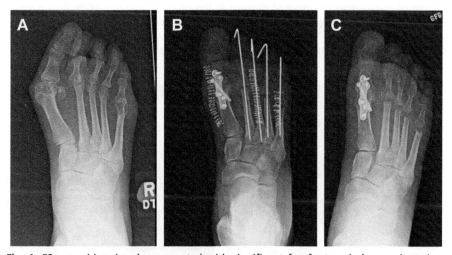

Fig. 4. 53-year-old male who presented with significant forefoot and abnormal erosions and bony cystic finding on plain film radiographs. After a laboratory workup, advanced imaging and orthopedic oncology consultation, the patient was found to be an undiagnosed Rheumatoid arthritis patient. After formal consultation with Rheumatology with medical therapy, the patient was deemed to be well controlled and surgery was undertaken using a 1st MTP arthrodesis, pan metatarsal head resection of the lesser metatarsal, and digital pinning. (*A*) Preoperative AP radiograph. (*B*) Immediate postoperative image and (*C*) 2-month postoperative weight bearing radiograph.

the first ray and allow for recreation of a normal metatarsal parabola. **Fig. 5** shows the void present after the removal of a synthetic cartilage hemi-graft (see **Fig. 5**). The void left from a small synthetic cartilage graft can be filled using autologous cancellous graft from the calcaneus or a small amount of allograft. **Fig. 6** shows an example of a failed synthetic cartilage graft converted to an arthrodesis (see **Fig. 6**). Standard fixation can be used when the bone void is small, but consider revision arthrodesis plates for larger voids and larger graft requirements (**Fig. 7**).

SURGICAL PEARLS

- Meticulous joint preparation with the use of indication specific or standard tools (ie, curettes, osteotomes) are a key component to optimal alignment and fusion rates
- Supplemental cancellous autograft from the calcaneus can be helpful in primary or revision cases
- Structural autograft can be obtained from the calcaneus, with care taken to avoid Iatrogenic fracture or injury. This location alleviates the need for iliac crest autograft and can reduce donor site morbidity
- Alignment of the interphalangeal joint of the hallux and the metatarsophalageanl joint fusion site can allow for optimal alignment, avoiding unnecessary varus, or valgus malposition
- Staple fixation can allow for less dissection, especially on the proximal phalanx, as well as avoiding any unnecessary prominence in patients with thinner skin envelopes

POSTOPERATIVE MANAGEMENT

The initial postoperative dressing applied in the operating room consists of a well-padded sterile dressing with a short leg compression dressing and posterior splint. Sutures are removed 10 to 14 days postop. Radiographs are taken at this visit to confirm appropriate alignment and hardware placement. The patient is placed in a full-length

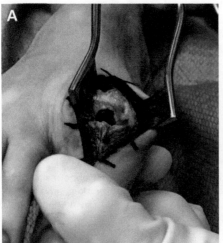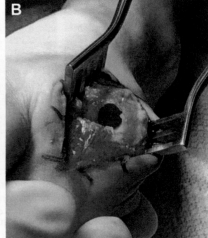

Fig. 5. (*A*) Failed synthetic cartilage implant and (*B*) bone void left from synthetic cartilage hemi-arthroplasty.

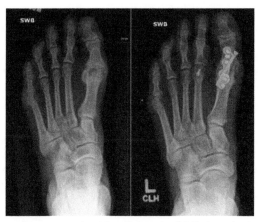

Fig. 6. Preoperative and postoperative AP radiograph of failed synthetic cartilage graft converted to an arthrodesis.

fracture (cam) walker and if the wound is stable, full heel touch weight-bearing with gentle forefoot pressure (weight of leg) to tolerance using crutch or walker assistance is encouraged. The patient is instructed to remove the boot several times per day to work on foot and ankle ROM exercises. Several studies have shown a high union rate with immediate weight-bearing after this technique. Berlet and Hyer reported 91%

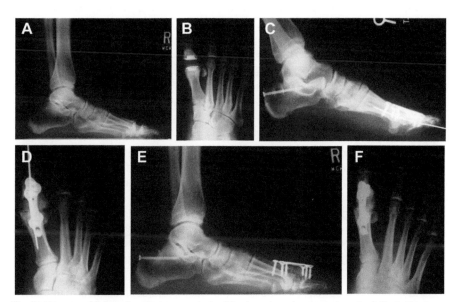

Fig. 7. 71-year-old female who presented with chronic pain secondary to failed silastic arthroplasty with aseptic osteolysis and grommet loosening of 1st MTP. The revision surgical plan included bulk calcaneal autograft for 1st MTP arthrodesis. The graft donor site is backfilled with size-matched allograft and fixated with a single fully threaded screw. Preoperative lateral and AP (A, B) imaging, as well as, initial postoperative (C, D) and 1-year follow-up imaging (E, F) demonstrating mature union at both the first MTP and donor graft site are noted.

clinical and radiographic union in 37 patients after immediate weight-bearing protocol for first MTP arthrodesis.[3] After sutures are removed, the patient may progress to full WB as tolerated in the boot. Radiographs are repeated at 6-weeks postop and patient may gradually transition back to a supportive shoe with orthotic support or carbon fiber insert when there is radiographic evidence of early consolidation. Patients are followed for 6 to 12-months postoperatively to ensure satisfactory outcome.

SUMMARY

The fusion of the 1st MTP is a safe, effective, and reproducible treatment of various indications of 1st MTP pathology including hallux valgus, hallux varus, failed MTP implant, revision surgery, and complex reconstruction. Types of fixation for surgical fusion have continued to evolve as the procedure has found more utility in the treatment of multiple pathologies of the first ray.

DISCLOSURE

Dr C. Hyer – consultant/IP from Stryker. Dr R. Brandão-is a consultant for Medline. Dr M. Prissel-no relevant conflicts to this article. Dr M. Dujela-no relevant conflicts to this article. Dr T. Langan-is a consultant for Medline and Artelon. Dr C. Fidler-no relevant conflicts to this article.

REFERENCES

1. Goucher NR, Coughlin MJ. Hallux metatarsophalangeal joint arthrodesis using dome-shaped reamers and dorsal plate fixation: a prospective study. Foot Ankle Int 2006;27(11):869–76.
2. Bennett GL, Sabetta J. First metatarsalphalangeal joint arthrodesis: evaluation of plate and screw fixation. Foot Ankle Int 2009;30(8):752–7.
3. Berlet GC, Hyer CF, Glover JP. A retrospective review of immediate weightbearing after first metatarsophalangeal joint arthrodesis. Foot Ankle Spec 2008;1:24–8.
4. Clutton H. The treatment of hallux valgus. St Thomas Rep 1894;22:1–12.
5. Rammelt S, Panzner I, Mittlmeier T. Metatarsophalangeal joint fusion: why and how? Foot Ankle Clin 2015;20:465–77.
6. Korim MT, Mahadevan D, Ghosh A, et al. Effect of joint pathology, surface preparation and fixation methods on union frequency after first metatarsophalangeal joint arthrodesis: a systematic review of the English literature. Foot Ankle Surg 2017;23:189–94.
7. Lacoste KL, Andrews NA, Ray J, et al. First metatarsophalangeal joint arthrodesis: a narrative review of fixation constructs and their evolution. Cureus 2021; 13(4):e14458.
8. Brodsky JW, Baum BS. Prospective gait analysis in patients with first metatarsophalangeal joint arthrodesis for hallux rigidus. Foot Ankle Int 2007;28(2):162–5.
9. Coughlin MJ, Abdo RV. Arthrodesis of the first metatarsophalangeal joint with Vitallium plate fixation. Foot Ankle Int 1994;15:18–28.
10. Hunt KJ, Ellington JK, Anderson RB, et al. Locked versus nonlocked plate fixation for hallux MTP arthrodesis. Foot Ankle Int 2011;32:704–9.
11. Frigg R. Locking compression plate (LCP). An osteosynthesis plate based on the dynamic compression plate and the point contact fixator (PC-Fix). Injury 2001; 32(Suppl 2):63–6.

12. Choudhary RK, Theruvil B, Taylor GR. First metatarsophalangeal joint arthrodesis: a new technique of internal fixation by using memory compression staples. J Foot Ankle Surg 2004;43:312–7.

13. Cronin JJ, Limbers JP, Kutty S, et al. Intermetatarsal angle after first metatarsophalangeal joint arthrodesis for hallux valgus. Foot Ankle Int 2006;27(2):104–9.

14. McKean RM, Bergin PF, Watson G, et al. Radiographic evaluation of intermetatarsal angle correction following first MTP joint arthrodesis for severe hallux valgus. Foot Ankle Int 2016;37(11):1183–6.

15. Dayton P, LoPiccolo J, Kiley J. Reduction of the intermetatarsal angle after first metatarsophalangeal joint arthrodesis in patients with moderate and severe metatarsus primus adductus. J Foot Ankle Surg 2002;41(5):316–9.

16. Sung W, Kluesner AJ, Irrgang J, et al. Radiographic outcomes following primary arthrodesis of the first metatarsophalangeal joint in hallux abductovalgus deformity. J Foot Ankle Surg 2010;49(5):446–51.

17. Dalat F, Cottalorda F, Fessy MH, et al. Does arthrodesis of the first metatarsophalangeal joint correct the intermetatarsal M1M2 angle? Analysis of a continuous series of 208 arthrodeses fixed with plates. Orthopaedics Traumatol Surg Res 2015;101(6):709–14.

18. Grimes JS, Coughlin MJ. First metatarsophalangeal joint arthrodesis as a treatment for failed hallux valgus surgery. Foot Ankle Int 2006;27(11):887–93.

19. Humbert JL, Bourbonniere C, Laurin CA. Metatarsophalangeal fusion for hallux valgus: indications and effect on the first metatarsal ray. Can Med Assoc J 1979;120(8):937.

20. Garras DN, Durinka JB, Bercik M, et al. Conversion arthrodesis for failed first metatarsophalangeal joint hemiarthroplasty. Foot Ankle Int 2013;34(9):1227–32.

21. Hecht PJ, Gibbons MJ, Wapner KL, et al. Arthrodesis of the first metatarsophalangeal joint to salvage failed silicone implant arthroplasty. Foot Ankle Int 1997;18(7):383–90.

22. Greisberg J. The failed first metatarsophalangeal joint implant arthroplasty. Foot Ankle Clin 2014;19(3):343–8.

Lesser Metatarsophalangeal Plantar Plate Repair

Christopher F. Hyer, DPM, MS, FACFAS[a],*, Devon Consul, DPM, BSN, AACFAS[b],
Jeffrey E. McAlister, DPM, FACFAS[c], James M. Cottom, DPM, FACFAS[d]

KEYWORDS

- Plantar plate injury • Lesser metatarsophalangeal joint instability
- Lesser toe deformity • Crossover toe

KEY POINTS

- Lesser MTP joint instability may be the result of plantar plate attentuation or an outright tear creating pain and instability.
- The lesser MTP joint plantar plate repair may be done via either a direct plantar approach or through a dorsal approach. The rationale for both techniques is discussed.
- A lesser metatarsal osteotomy is sometimes used as a treatment and as a means of access for the dorsal approach repair.

INTRODUCTION

Lesser toe plantar plate injuries at the metatarsophalangeal (MTP) joint are a common source of metatarsalgia. Chronic pain with weight-bearing is the common presentation of lesser toe instability.[1,2] A variety of surgical procedures have been proposed to straighten the toe and reduce plantar pressure and pain. Although the surgical management of the dorsally subluxed second MTP is difficult, with sometimes unpredictable long-term results. The most routinely used procedures use straightening of the digit via arthroplasty or arthrodesis, soft tissue rebalancing of the MTP, flexor tendon transfer, metatarsal head resection, or metatarsal osteotomy.

However, none of these surgical procedures have consistently provided satisfactory postoperative outcomes alone. Achieving a pain free, neutral position of the toe often requires an in-depth understanding of both the soft tissue and osseous structures affected and using a combination of surgical options best suited to each individual.

[a] Board Certified, Foot & Ankle Reconstructive Surgery, Advanced Foot & Ankle Reconstruction, Ofac, American College of Foot and Ankle Surgeons, American College of Foot and Ankle Surgeons, Foot & Ankle Surgery, Masters Science, Clinical Research, Drexel School of Medicine, 350 West Wilson Bridge Road Suite 200, Worthington, OH 43085, USA; [b] Orthopedic Foot and Ankle Center, 350 West Wilson Bridge Road Suite 200, Worthington, OH 43085, USA; [c] Phoenix Foot and Ankle Institute, 7301 East 2nd Street Suite 206, Scottsdale, AZ 85251, USA; [d] Florida Orthopedic Foot and Ankle Center, Florida Orthopedic Foot & Ankle Center, 1630 South Tuttle Avenue Suite A, Sarasota, FL 34239, USA
* Corresponding author.
E-mail address: hyercf@orthofootankle.com

Clin Podiatr Med Surg 39 (2022) 167–185
https://doi.org/10.1016/j.cpm.2021.11.008
0891-8422/22/© 2021 Elsevier Inc. All rights reserved.

podiatric.theclinics.com

In this article, the authors present a comprehensive stepwise approach to diagnosing and treating plantar plate injuries.

HISTORY

Lesser MTP joint instability has challenged surgeons for decades. Coughlin and colleagues first described crossover toe deformity in 1987, with the second MTP joint being the most commonly affected.[1,3] Evolutions in the nomenclature have been experienced over that same time; hammertoe, crossover toe, metatarsalgia, predislocation syndrome, and dislocated toe have all be used in describing instability as it relates to the structures of the second MTP joint. For more than 25 years, the management of lesser MTP instability has been characterized by indirect repairs of the deformity using soft tissue release, extensor or flexor tendon transfer, and periarticular osteotomy.[4–7]

The causes of lesser toe subluxation and dislocation are still unclear but are probably multifactorial. Risk factors such as acute trauma, high-fashion shoe wear, rheumatoid arthritis, and other various inflammatory conditions have all been linked to metatarsalgia and lesser MTP instability.[5–7] Although more recently the clinical and surgical understanding of lesser MTP pathoanatomy has advanced with a greater recognition to both the osseous and soft tissue derangement present. Due to this greater understanding, substantial progress has been made in the development of improved surgical techniques and instrumentation.

DEFINITION

The plantar plate is a fibrocartilaginous structure which is a dorsal restraint to the MTP. Deformity occurs when the plantar plate is torn or attenuated. Crossover toe and MTP instability often occur with multiplane deformity, most commonly with dorsal contracture of the second toe and medial drift over the Hallux.[2]

BACKGROUND

A thorough patient history and physical examination is always performed. Discussions related to prior history of trauma, inappropriate shoe gear, and concomitant deformity should be had. Additionally, an understanding of the patient's surgical history and medical conditions is also important.

Clinically, in both the acute and chronic setting patients typically present with complaints of pain in the ball of their foot, with or without concern for hammertoe development. It is imperative with digital and forefoot pathology to assess patients' feet in a loaded and unloaded position. A gait analysis should also be explored to assess forefoot and hindfoot position during ambulation. Foot architecture should be evaluated and documented as a pes planovalgus foot structure predisposes itself to the injury of the lesser MTP joint. Focusing on the lesser MTP deformity most commonly involves attention to the second MTP. The associated Hallux Valgus if present should also be documented.

In addition to the initial examination, a standard series of weight-bearing radiographs should be obtained. Anteroposterior radiographs typically demonstrate transverse plane deformity of the proximal phalanx of the metatarsal and will give the surgeon better detail as to procedural selection. The authors do recommend advanced imaging if there is a concern for plantar plate tear. Ultrasound and magnetic resonance imaging are valuable in determining the status of the plantar plate and associated structures. MRI can also be used to identify additional pathology related to the involved articular margins of the MTP joint and bone. The surgeon can then plan surgical intervention with an appropriate understanding of the involved pathoanatomy.

DISCUSSION

Regarding the surgical techniques, an appropriate recommendation for a particular surgical approach remains patient specific and based on the surgeon's preference. Surgeons across disciplines have identified the plantar plate as a source of lesser MTP pain, leading to deformity. A multitude of surgical procedures has been proposed over the past decades to treat injuries of the plantar plate including tendon transfers, metatarsal osteotomies, dorsal soft tissue balancing, plantar soft tissue repair, MTP arthrodesis, and MTP arthroplasty. Previously a reluctance to operate on the plantar aspect of the forefoot led to techniques focused on dorsal approaches in conjunction with metatarsal osteotomies to directly visualize lesser MTP pathology. Overtime, techniques have evolved as surgeons' comfort levels grew leading to both dorsal and plantar surgical approaches for plantar plate repair. Primary repair of the plantar plate via a plantar forefoot approach is now a viable and effective method for treating instability and pathology of the plantar plate.

The purpose of this article remains to provide surgeons with descriptions of surgical approaches for the treatment of plantar plate injuries. Whether electing for a dorsal approach to repair, or the plantar technique for repair, surgical pearls allow for foot and ankle surgeons to adequately visualize the plantar structures. These exposures and direct visualization of pathology have afforded an opportunity for dramatic correction of lesser MTP instability and injury.

Techniques

Direct plantar plate repair technique: plantar approach

Patients are typically on the operating room table in the supine position. An ipsilateral extremity bump is placed under the hip to orient the extremity in an upright position. General anesthesia with a preoperative popliteal block is performed. A thigh tourniquet is applied and inflated to the surgeon's preference. A mini C-arm is used and positioned on the same side of the surgical extremity. Appropriate prepping of the operative extremity is performed to the level of the tourniquet. Esmarch exsanguination is often performed to reduce the incidence of intraoperative bleeding which may affect the visualization of pertinent plantar anatomy.

Typical instrumentation includes appropriate suture material for collateral ligament and plantar plate repair. Sagittal saw and power drivers are used as needed for additional osseous procedures that are performed at the time of soft tissue repair. The authors prefer small cannulated or twist-off partial thread screws for fixation, 2.0/2.5/2.7 mm for metatarsal osteotomies. The soft tissues structures including plantar plate are traditionally repaired using 2 to 0 nonabsorbable or 0 absorbable sutures. The hammertoe when present is corrected per the surgeon's preferred method. In cases of plantar plate repair using on-lay grafting or anchor placement, the surgeon may elect to pin the hammertoe and MTP joint into a slightly plantarflexed neutral position to aid in healing and protection of the soft tissue repair during postoperative recovery.

Step 1: Intraoperative direct plantar approach via 2.5 cm linear or curvilinear incision is performed and provides direct adequate visualization of the plantar plate. The direct plantar approach also reduces the necessity to perform concomitant metatarsal osteotomies for the visualization of the plantar plate (**Fig. 1**).

Step 2: Intraoperative photograph of the incision carried out on the plantar aspect of the foot beneath the associated MTP joint and distal metatarsal. Dissection is carried

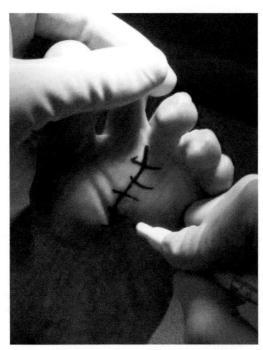

Fig. 1. Step 1: Intraoperative direct plantar approach via 2.5 cm linear or curvilinear incision is performed and provides direct adequate visualization of the plantar plate. The direct plantar approach also reduces the necessity to perform concomitant metatarsal osteotomies for visualization of the plantar plate.

deep through subcutaneous adipose tissues until the flexor tendon sheath is visualized (**Fig. 2**).

Step 3: A linear flexor tendon sheath incision is then performed, typically starting at the most distal extent (base of phalanx) and extending proximally for adequate exposure of the long and short flexor tendons. In profound multiplanar deformity, the tendons may be subluxed medially or laterally (**Fig. 3**).

Step 4: Intraoperative photo with Weitlander retractor (small) used to split the flexor tendons to the medial and lateral aspects of the incision, providing direct exposure of the plantar plate and associated pathology.

Step 5: The surgeon will more often find diseased and attenuated plantar plate soft tissues, in other instances complete tearing of the plantar plate is encountered (demonstrated with the placement of the freer elevator). Excision of the damaged plantar plate tissues is then performed via sharp dissection with a no15 blade.

Step 6: (Option) Transverse plane deformities can often be addressed at the time of repair by removal of nonviable soft tissue via wedge resection of the involved tissues, commonly 2 mm of wedge resection is needed to correct transverse plane angulation (**Fig. 4**).

Step 7: In repairs whereby there are available healthy plantar plate tissues at the base of the proximal phalanx a direct apposition and repair of the plantar plate is accomplished with selected suture material and pants over vest suture technique.

Step 8: When more severe pathology is encountered additional implants and instrumentation may be used to appropriately repair the plantar plate. Intraoperative imaging demonstrates placement of a suture anchor into the base of the proximal phalanx

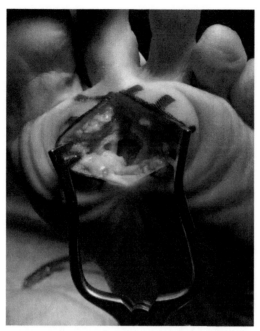

Fig. 2. Step 2: Intraoperative photograph of the incision carried out on the plantar aspect of the foot beneath the associated metatarsophalangeal joint and distal metatarsal. Dissection is carried deep through subcutaneous adipose tissues until the flexor tendon sheath is visualized.

with synthetic graft-on-lay to reapproximate proximal plantar plate tissues to the base of the proximal phalanx. Repair is performed with the toe manually held in slight plantarflexion and neutral MTP alignment. The final resting position of the digit should be slightly plantarflexed when compared with adjacent digits.

Postoperative image of the healed plantar approach incision. Closure is accomplished with deep absorbable suture placement. The skin is repaired with a horizontal mattress technique allowing for the eversion of the skin edges (**Fig. 5**).

Postoperative weight-bearing anteroposterior postoperative radiograph demonstrating multiplane correction of the second MTP deformity. Neutral positional correction of the lesser MTP joint is accomplished (**Fig. 6**).

Postoperative weight-bearing lateral postoperative radiograph demonstrating multiplane correction of the second MTP deformity. Neutral positional correction of the lesser MTP joint is accomplished (**Fig. 7**).

DORSAL APPROACH WITH OBLIQUE METATARSAL OSTEOTOMY

Hallux valgus is addressed first when present, with the procedure at the discretion of the surgeon. Requisite reduction of 1 to 2 intermetatarsal deformity with a hallux valgus angle 0 to 15° is necessary. Once the first ray is in normal anatomic alignment, attention is then directed to the affected lesser MTP(s). If multiple digits are being corrected, start with the most medial. Digital contracture is addressed first, usually with proximal interphalangeal joint (PIPJ) preparation for arthrodesis through a dorsal longitudinal incisional approach. Definitive fixation with a Kirschner wire or an intramedullary implant may be placed now or delayed until the repair of plantar plate (if needed).

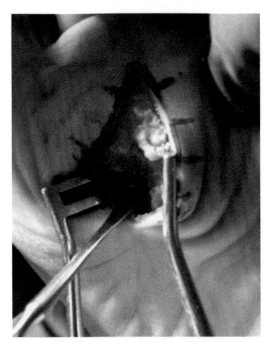

Fig. 3. Step 3: A linear flexor tendon sheath incision is then performed, typically starting at the most distal extent (base of phalanx) and extending proximally for adequate exposure of the long and short flexor tendons. In profound multiplanar deformity the tendons may be subluxed medially or laterally.

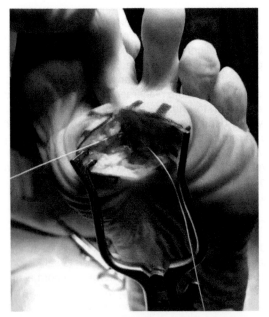

Fig. 4. Step 4: Intraoperative photo with Weitlander retractor (small) used to split the flexor tendons to the medial and lateral aspects of the incision, providing direct exposure of the plantar plate and associated pathology.

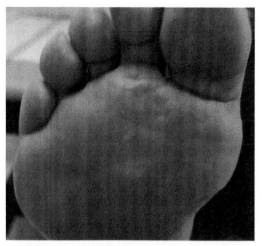

Fig. 5. Postoperative image of the healed plantar approach incision.

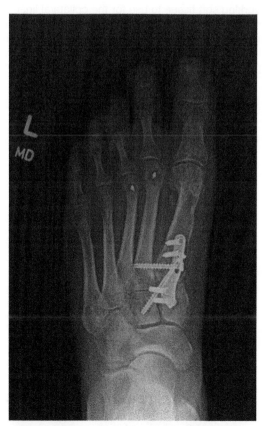

Fig. 6. Postoperative weight-bearing anteroposterior postoperative radiograph demonstrating the multiplane correction of the second metatarsophalangeal deformity. Neutral positional correction of the lesser metatarsophalangeal joint is accomplished.

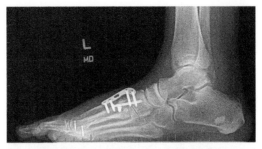

Fig. 7. Postoperative weight-bearing lateral postoperative radiograph demonstrating multiplane correction of the second metatarsophalangeal deformity. Neutral positional correction of the lesser metatarsophalangeal joint is accomplished.

The incision is lengthened proximally in a curvilinear fashion to gain exposure to the MTP to prevent inadvertent dorsal skin (and digital) contracture. One can also make 2 separate incisions—over the PIPJ and separately just proximal to the lesser MTP. The extensor digitorum longus is opened in "Z" fashion to facilitate later repair in a lengthened state. Perform a dorsal transverse capsulotomy at the MTP and transect the medial and lateral collateral ligaments and dorsal capsule midsubstance. This allows appropriate working soft tissue to use for the collateral ligament repair.

At this point, perform the metatarsal osteotomy (**Fig. 8**). With the medial deviation of the digit, make the osteotomy in an oblique fashion to shorten and realign the toe (**Figs. 9** and **10**). The osteotomy is oriented from dorsal to plantar, perpendicular to the weight-bearing surface of the foot so that with the translation of the cut from

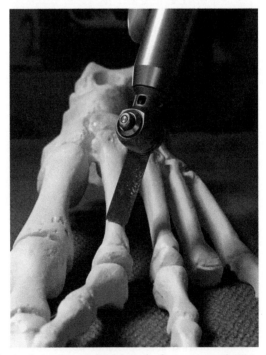

Fig. 8. Metatarsal osteotomy perpendicular to the lesser toe and 45° to the weightbearing surface of the foot.

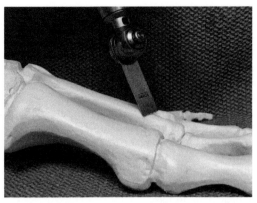

Fig. 9. Note the orientation of the saw blade and proximity to the adjacent articular cartilage. This will allow extraarticular screws to be placed appropriately.

medial to lateral (or vice versa, depending on deformity), no dorsal or plantar shifting
will occur. The cut is oriented from distal lateral to proximal medial most commonly
(with a medial crossover toe). If there is lateral deviation of the digit, the osteotomy
is in the opposite direction. Of note, the osteotomy is approximately 45° to the long
axis of the metatarsal and is started just proximal (0.5 cm) to the articular cartilage
of the metatarsal head, within the neck, and is completed in the distal diaphysis.
The intention is to have a large enough capital fragment for fixation without having
to violate the articular surface. This will allow the surgeon to translate the capital

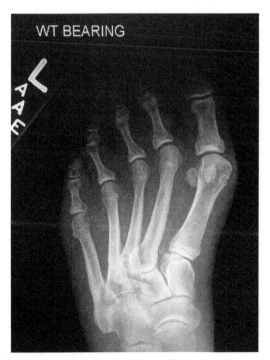

Fig. 10. Severe hallux valgus deformity with lesser MTP lateral transverse plane deformity
without severe digital contractures.

fragment medially (or laterally) and proximally to the desired level. The surgeon can also translate dorsally 1–2 mm if desired to off-load the plantar plate. This osteotomy has now been introduced as the B-Mac (Bouche-McAlister) metatarsal osteotomy.

After performing the osteotomy, translate the capital fragment to realign the toe to a rectus position, usually a minimum of one-third the width of the metatarsal. Temporarily fixate the capital fragment with a small Kirschner wire and be sure the toe has shifted in the appropriate position. It may be necessary to place the Kirschner wire through the PIPJ for the stability of the toe at this time. After confirming the correct position, fixate the capital fragment with either a threaded 0.062″ Kirschner wire or small screw(s) (1.5 mm – 2.5 mm) perpendicular to the osteotomy, distal to proximal, or proximal to distal. One or 2 points of fixation may be used. Care should be taken not to violate the articular surface of the metatarsal head or to place fixation protruding from the plantar surface that may damage the plantar plate. The length of screw or Kirschner wire is typically near 16 mm.

Confirm correction on intraoperative fluoroscopy. We have found that a medial or lateral shift of at least one-third to one-half the width of the metatarsal is required. Take care not to over-correct, as this osteotomy is very powerful (**Figs. 10** and **11** – lateral deviation) (**Figs. 12** and **13** – medial deviation). Close the attenuated collateral ligaments and capsule with a nonabsorbable suture in the mid- to plantar aspect of the joint so as not to inadvertently cause a dorsal contracture.

At this juncture, a small circle tapered needle is used to place 2 sutures in the proximal aspect of the plantar plate just below the metatarsal head. Next, 2 drill holes are placed into the base of the proximal phalanx with a Kirschner wire through the base of the proximal phalanx. Typically, nonabsorbable sutures are used so as to retain the

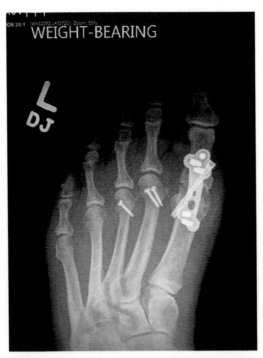

Fig. 11. Status-post 2 months lesser metatarsal osteotomies and collateral ligament reconstruction and first MTP fusion.

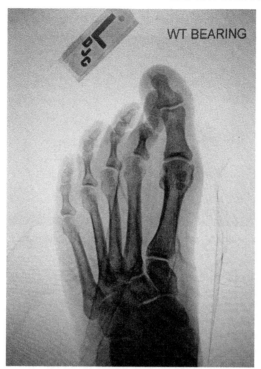

Fig. 12. Mild increase in hallux valgus angle with medial deviation of lesser metatarsophalangeal joints 2 and 3 with digital contractures.

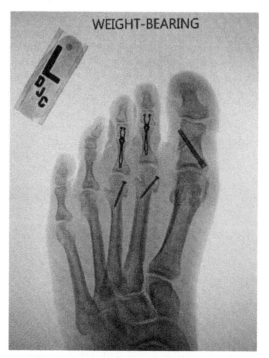

Fig. 13. Status-post 6 weeks. Corrective proximal phalanx osteotomy and medial translational osteotomies of the lesser metatarsals with intramedullary fixation of the hammertoes.

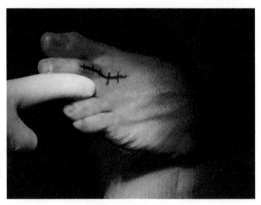

Fig. 14. Dorsal incision slightly curved over the metatarsophalangeal joint.

strength and integrity of the construct. The digit is held in a slightly plantarflexed attitude while the sutures are approximated. Proceed to repair the extensor digitorum longus in a lengthened position.

Postoperatively, the patient typically bears weight immediately in a controlled ankle motion (CAM) walker fracture boot for 4 to 6 weeks until radiographic healing occurs and then transitions to a supportive shoe. The lesser digits are splinted in the appropriate position (if no k-wires present) for 6 weeks (see **Fig. 13**).

PLANTAR PLATE REPAIR WITH EXTENSIVE TISSUE DAMAGE

To perform this technique, the patient is placed in a supine position with a well-padded ipsilateral thigh tourniquet inflated to 300 mm Hg. A 4 cm slightly curved incision is placed over the affected metatarsal phalangeal joint (MTP) and extended out to the PIPJ. This is done to prevent postoperative scarring of the extensor tendon which could lead to a dorsal contracture of the digit (**Fig. 14**). Next, the extensor tendons are retracted medially or laterally and a linear capsulotomy is made over the joint.

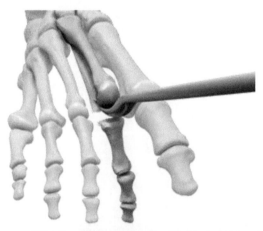

Fig. 15. A McGlamry elevator is used to release the proximal plantar plate inferior to the metatarsal head/neck. Keep McGlamry in-line with MT shaft and refrain from releasing accessory collateral ligaments from the metatarsal head.

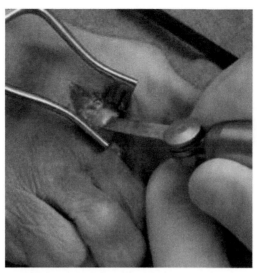

Fig. 16. A Weil osteotomy is performed starting 2mm–3 mm below the superior articular surface and parallel to the weight-bearing surface of the foot.

Next, the collateral ligaments at the base of the proximal phalanx are released and a McGlamry elevator is used to release the proximal plantar plate inferior to the metatarsal head/neck (**Fig. 15**). A Weil osteotomy is then performed starting 2–3 mm below the superior aspect of the articular surface of the metatarsal head and should be made

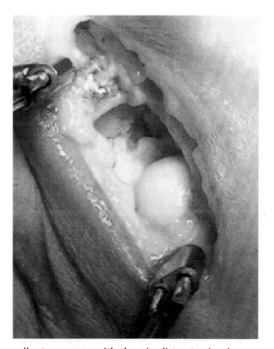

Fig. 17. Note the excellent exposure with the pin distractor in place.

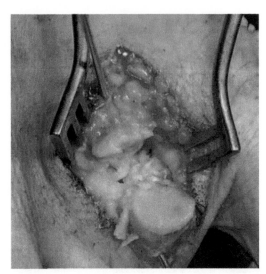

Fig. 18. Note the extensive degeneration and fraying of the plantar plate.

parallel to the weight-bearing surface of the foot (**Fig. 16**). A k-wire is then used to provisionally hold the Weil osteotomy in its final position and it is recommended to place this wire a little off-center of the metatarsal bone to allow for later drilling for the plantar plate repair. Another k-wire is then placed centrally into the base of the proximal phalanx of the digit. A pin distractor is then placed over the initial k-wires and the joint

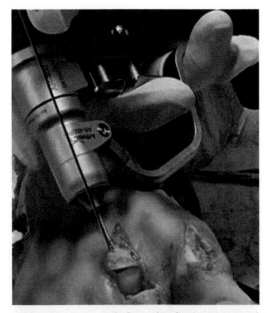

Fig. 19. The metatarsal head is temporarily fixated in final position with the initial k-wire, a second guidewire for a 2.5 mm drill is placed dorsally at least 5 mm proximal and centrally on the metatarsal and aimed toward the inferior central aspect of the metatarsal.

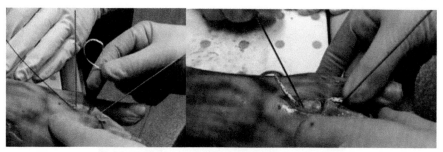

Fig. 20. The suture tape is double loaded and pulled proximally through the drill hole with a suture passer and can be clamped with a small hemostat to keep the suture tape from pulling back through the bone tunnel.

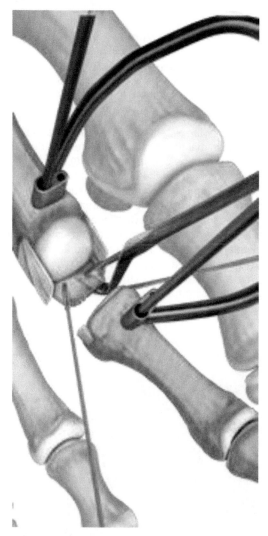

Fig. 21. The plantar plate mobilized the CPR Viper (Arthrex, Naples, FL) is placed into the joint and the plantar plate is grasped medially and laterally spaced out 3 mm to 5 mm with the distal ends of the suture tape.

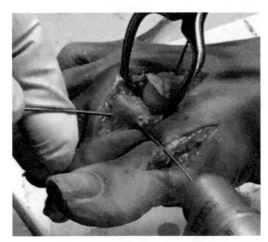

Fig. 22. The k-wire in the proximal phalanx is used as a "joystick" and the proximal phalanx is plantar flexed to obtain access for k-wire to be placed bicortically through the proximal phalanx. This wire can be placed either medial to lateral or from dorsal to plantar.

distracted to access the plantar plate (**Fig. 17**). At this time the plantar plate can be evaluated and if there is minimal healthy tissue or extensive degeneration, then a suture tape augmented repair can be performed (**Fig. 18**).

First, the remaining attachments of the plantar plate are sharply resected from the base of the proximal phalanx and any degenerated tissue is removed to reduce inflammatory pain postoperatively. Next, with the metatarsal head already held in final position with the initial k-wire, a second guidewire for a 2.5 mm drill is placed dorsally at least 5 mm proximal and centrally on the metatarsal and aimed toward the inferior central aspect of the metatarsal (**Fig. 19**). The cannulated 2.5 mm drill is then used and drilled over the guidewire. Then a suture passer is placed through the prepared bone tunnel in the metatarsal and the sharp end of the passer is pushed through the plantar plate remnant. Using forceps with teeth and pulling the remnant plantar

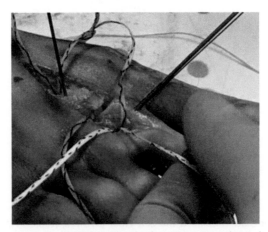

Fig. 23. A suture passer is then used to shuttle the suture tape through the proximal phalanx from lateral to medial with one end and medial to lateral with the other.

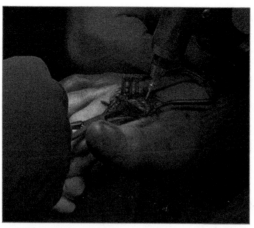

Fig. 24. Fixation of the Weil osteotomy before tensioning of the suture tape. It is recommended to use 2 screws for this for rotational stability.

plate distally makes this quite easy to accomplish. Next, the suture tape is double loaded and pulled proximally through the drill hole and held with a small hemostat (**Fig. 20**). With the plantar plate mobilized the CPR Viper (Arthrex, Naples, FL) is placed into the joint and the plantar plate is grasped medially and laterally spaced out 3 mm to 5 mm with the distal ends of the suture tape (**Fig. 21**). At this time the pin distractor is removed and the k-wire in the proximal phalanx is used as a "joystick" and the proximal phalanx is plantar flexed to obtain access for k-wire to be placed bicortically though the proximal phalanx. This wire can be placed either from dorsal to plantar or medial to lateral depending on if there is a transverse plane deformity that needs to be addressed (**Fig. 22**). A 2.5 mm cannulated drill bit is used to drill the bicortical tunnel in the phalanx. A suture passer is then used to shuttle the suture tape through the proximal phalanx and clamped with a hemostat for later tensioning (**Fig. 23**). Next, the Weil osteotomy is fixated with 2 small snap-off screws for rotational stability (**Fig. 24**). Make sure the proximal end of the suture tape in the metatarsal is still

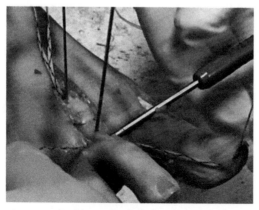

Fig. 25. Secure the suture tape in the proximal phalanx with a 3 mm × 8 mm PEEK Tenodesis Screw (Arthrex, Naples, FL) into the proximal phalanx.

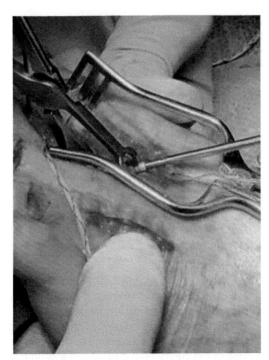

Fig. 26. Impact the base of the proximal phalanx into the metatarsal head and with 25 to 30 of plantarflexion, simulate weight-bearing and make sure the digit is in the final desired position. Pull back on the looped end of the suture tape in the metatarsal, cut the looped end and separate the suture tape medially and laterally and insert another 3 mm × 8 mm PEEK Tenodesis Screw (Arthrex, Naples, FL) into the metatarsal.

clamped with a hemostat and secure the suture tape in the proximal phalanx with a 3 mm × 8 mm PEEK Tenodesis Screw (Arthrex, Naples, FL) into the proximal phalanx **(Fig. 25)**. This will essentially lock in the suture tape in the proximal phalanx. With the base of the proximal phalanx impacted into the metatarsal head and with 25 to 30° of plantarflexion, simulate weight-bearing and make sure the digit is in the final desired position. Pull back on the looped end of the suture tape in the metatarsal, cut the looped end and separate the suture tape medially and laterally and insert another 3 mm × 8 mm PEEK Tenodesis Screw (Arthrex, Naples, FL) into the metatarsal between the suture tape ends **(Fig 26)**. Then cut all ends of the suture tape flush with the bone. Routine closure is performed, and the patient is placed in a compression dressing and postoperative shoe or short cam walker boot for 10 to 14 days and is allowed to weight bear as tolerated. Sutures are removed at 10 to 14 days, physical therapy is started as well as transition to regular shoe gear once the soft tissue and bone healing are ready.

DISCLOSURES

The authors have nothing to disclose.

REFERENCES

1. Coughlin MJ. Crossover second toe deformity. Foot Ankle 1987;8:29–39.

2. Hyer CF, Berlet GC, Philbin TM, et al. Essential foot and ankle surgical techniques: a multidisciplinary approach. Springer 2019;57–68.
3. Nery C, Coughlin MJ, Baumfeld D, et al. Lesser metatarsophalangeal joint instability: prospective evaluation and repair of plantar plate and capsular insufficiency. Foot Ankle Int 2012;33:301–11.
4. Coughlin MJ. Subluxation and dislocation of the second metatarsophalangeal joint. Orthop Clin North Am 1989;20:535–51.
5. Haddad SL, Sabbagh RC, Resch S, et al. Results of flexor-to extensor and extensor brevis tendon transfer for correction of the crossover second toe deformity. Foot Ankle Int 1999;20:781–8.
6. Myerson MS, Jung HG. The role of toe flexor-to-extensor transfer in correcting metatarsophalangeal joint instability of the second toe. Foot Ankle Int 2005;26:675–9.
7. Ford LA, Collins KB, Christensen JC. Stabilization of the subluxed second metatarsophalangeal joint: flexor tendon transfer versus primary repair of the plantar plate. J Foot Ankle Surg 1998;37:217–22.

Lapidus Arthrodesis

Michael D. Dujela, DPM[a],*, Travis Langan, DPM[b],
James M. Cottom, DPM[c], William T. DeCarbo, DPM[d], Jeffrey E. McAlister, DPM[e],
Christopher F. Hyer, DPM, MS[f]

KEYWORDS

- Lapidus • Hallux valgus • Midfoot instability • Tarsometatarsal joint • Bunion
- Hypermobility first ray

KEY POINTS

- Accurate evaluation of the preoperative deformity is imperative to choose the correct surgical procedure that provides appropriate alignment of the first ray.
- Adequate release at the tarsometatarsal joint and metatarsophalangeal joint including the metatarsal sesamoid ligament allows for frontal plane correction, which is key in triplane realignment of hallux valgus deformities.
- Maintenance of first ray length via curettage joint preparation techniques is crucial.
- Various fixation constructs exist; however, plate and screw combinations assist in allowing early weight-bearing, return to function, and reduced risk of nonunion.
- Fixation constructs should include intermetatarsal and/or first metatarsal to intermediate cuneiform screw fixation to stabilize the medial column, prevent late diastasis, and recurrence of the deformity.

INTRODUCTION

Hallux abductovalgus (HAV) is a common, complex, and challenging deformity that foot and ankle surgeons face. More than 100 types of operations have been described for management. In 1934, Paul Lapidus expanded on the work of his predecessors Albrecht and Truslow and described an arthrodesis technique involving preparation of the first tarsometatarsal joint (TMT) as well as the space between the first and second metatarsal bases for enhanced stability.[1,2] Significant shortening of the first ray resulted via aggressive saw resection, and fixation

[a] Washington Orthopaedic Center, 1900 Cooks Hill Road, Centralia, WA 98532, USA; [b] Carle Clinic Orthopedics and Sports Medicine, 2300 S 1st Street, Champaign, IL, USA; [c] Florida Orthopedic Foot and Ankle Center, 1630 S Tuttle Avenue, Suite A, Sarasota, FL 34239, USA; [d] Foot and Ankle Division, St. Clair Medical Group, 3928 Washington Road. Ste 270, Pittsburgh, PA 15317, USA; [e] Phoenix Foot and Ankle Institute, 7301 E 2nd Street, Suite. 206, Scottsdale, AZ 85085, USA; [f] Orthopedic Foot and Ankle Center, 350 W Wilson Bridge Road Suite 200, Worthington, OH 43085, USA
* Corresponding author.
E-mail address: michaeldujela@yahoo.com

Clin Podiatr Med Surg 39 (2022) 187–206
https://doi.org/10.1016/j.cpm.2021.11.009
0891-8422/22/© 2021 Elsevier Inc. All rights reserved.

was insufficient using exclusively suture to stabilize the repair; this was complicated by the fact that postoperative management involved early weight-bearing
potentially resulting in malunion or nonunion. Various iterations over the past
90 years have been reported, with rigid internal fixation and early return to functional activity being the universally accepted approach in modern times. Over
the past several years at our institution, techniques have evolved from primarily internal screw fixation to now performing a curettage joint preparation technique
with crossing screws combined with locking plates. In our recent case series evaluating the results of this technique, the union rate was 97%.[3,4] This construct allows early return to function while minimizing risk of complications such as
arthrofibrosis and deep venous thrombosis.

Accurate evaluation of the preoperative deformity is imperative to choose the correct surgical procedure that provides appropriate alignment of the first ray. In addition
to a cosmetic outcome in the eyes of the patient, anatomic reduction and stability of
the first ray that results in excellent function with durable long-term outcomes is imperative. Until recently the terms hypermobility of the TMT, metatarsus primus varus, and
valgus alignment of the hallux have not addressed triplanar deformity.[5,6] To achieve
reliable long-term results, it is essential to understand and address anatomic deformity
reduction in all 3 cardinal planes.[7–9] Residual planar deformity often leads to results
that are unsatisfactory for both the patient and the surgeon and increases the risk
of recurrence.

Restoration of the anatomic "tripod" of the foot via a modern approach to a first TMT
arthrodesis is a valuable tool to assist in restoring medial column stability and in many
cases hindfoot deformities.

CLINICAL EVALUATION

Patients often present to foot and ankle surgeons with first metatarsophalangeal joint
(MTP) pain or pain from direct shoe pressure over the prominence. In addition to pain
with activity and ill-fitting shoes, patients also complain of the unsightliness from a
cosmetic perspective.

A thorough history and physical examination is performed. It is important to assess
whether there is any history of trauma or arthritic change of the first MTP joint or pain to
the second MTP or plantar plate. An important consideration is whether there is a history or physical findings consistent with neuropathy, which may increase the risk of
nonunion therefore warranting consideration of graft or orthobiologics; this may also
impact the choice of fixation.

The history should elicit whether pain is present with range of motion of the joint.
Significant pain, limitation of first MTP motion, and radiographic features consistent
with degenerative arthritis are relative contraindications for TMT joint fusion. It is
also important to assess the degree of dorsiflexion and plantarflexion, quality of range
of motion, as well as plantar MTP tenderness, which can indicate metatarsal-
sesamoid arthritic disease. The hallux interphalangeal joint and MTP should be free
of arthritic change when considering fusion of the TMT joint.

TMT joint range of motion is assessed for hypermobility and as in all aspects of the
examination, compared with the contralateral side for any asymmetry.[6,10–12] Evaluation of the second MTP for pain, edema, or instability is important. A plantar localized
callus may be a clue to overload.

Weight-bearing static analysis is performed to assess for associated deformity or
malalignment including forefoot and hindfoot. Gait analysis is performed to assess

function. In closed kinetic chain the hallux deformity, lesser toe deformities, as well as hindfoot and midfoot position can be assessed.[5]

IMAGING

The typical radiographic angles used when evaluating HAV deformity are the hallux abductus angle (HAA), the intermetatarsal angle (IMA), the tibial sesamoid position (TSP), and proximal and distal articular set angles. Recently an additional parameter termed the "lateral round sign" was described by Okuda and colleagues,[13] which evaluates frontal plane rotation of the first metatarsal. Valgus rotation of the first metatarsal results in radiographic appearance of the lateral edge of the first metatarsal head, which is not normally seen.[13]

The most common angles used to evaluate HAV deformity on a weight-bearing anteroposterior (AP) radiograph are the HAA (hallux abductus angle) and IMA (intermetatarsal angle). This is a consistent method to help determine the magnitude of the deformity; however, this is a 2-dimensional assessment and lacks the ability to assess the frontal plane rotation of the first metatarsal.[14–16] To determine the frontal plane rotation, the TSP and the "lateral round sign" become critical. Historically, it was thought that the sesamoids sublux from their groove and crista under the head of the first metatarsal. Recent publications have shown that the sesamoids remain in their original position and the transverse plane drift of the medial head of the first metatarsal and frontal plane rotation of the first metatarsal combine to give the radiographic appearance of sesamoid subluxation.[8,17,18] Another important radiographic finding to evaluate the frontal plane deformity of the first metatarsal is the "lateral round sign." With frontal plane rotation of the first metatarsal the lateral and plantar portion of the first metatarsal head creates a rounded appearance of the lateral metatarsal head. This rotation accentuates valgus position of the hallux.[8,13,17–19]

Radiographic evaluation is typically done with the standard 4-view weight-bearing radiographs, which include AP, lateral, medial oblique, and sesamoid axial views. It is often necessary to evaluate the hindfoot and ankle to ensure accurate assessment of the radiographic alignment of the foot and ankle. The AP radiographc view can assess the transverse plane deformity by evaluating both the IMA and HAA. The lateral radiograph is used to evaluate the sagittal plane alignment and deformity. To evaluate the frontal plane both the AP view to assess the lateral round sign and sesamoid axial view are used. On the AP view the medial sesamoid position is evaluated in relation to the bisection of the first metatarsal axis.[20] The grading system is 1 to 7 with displacement being viewed as a position of 5 or greater.[21] The sesamoid axial view is a reliable way to assess malposition and frontal plane rotation of the sesamoids and first metatarsal.[22] The AP view also evaluates the IMA and the HAA. The angles measured on all 4 radiographic views have historically been used to determine which of the more than 100 published surgical procedures for hallux valgus correction should be used when combined with clinical examination. In 2002, Pentikainen and colleagues[23] described the parameters of measurement and ranges of deformity to determine appropriate procedure selection. The investigators suggest that a distal metatarsal osteotomy is suitable for correction of a mild increased IMA of less than 9° to 11° and moderate angle increase of 11° to 16°. In severe deformities of greater than 16°, a proximal osteotomy or TMT joint fusion is indicated. Hatch and colleagues[24] proposed a new classification and evaluation process composed of 4 classifications, which identify the radiographic presence of frontal plane rotation with or without degenerative joint disease of the first MTP and sesamoid complex. Based on these findings, surgical management is via metatarsal osteotomy, triplane correction with TMT fusion, second and third TMT correction with fusion, or first MTP fusion. This paradigm shift may offer more appropriate procedure choices and offer the patient more consistent long-term outcomes.

TECHNIQUES
Lapidus: Orthopedic Foot and Ankle Center Technique

Cross screw to intermediate cuneiform with dorsal medial plate or staple fixation, optional added first to second intermetatarsal screw
The addition of a screw from the base of the first metatarsal to the base of the second metatarsal can help achieve deformity correction and add additional stability.[3,4] Recent studies have shown that the addition of this screw can improve intermetatarsal angular correction and allow for maintenance of correction.[3]

Technique
The patient is placed in a supine position with a well-padded ipsilateral thigh tourniquet. Next, a 4-cm incision is planned over the medial aspect of the first TMT (**Fig. 1**) Subperiosteal dissection is performed to expose the base of the first metatarsal and medial cuneiform. The insertion of the tibialis anterior tendon is protected. A pin distractor is used to distract the joint after release of the plantar ligaments, and appropriate joint preparation is completed (**Fig. 2**).

Joint preparation is performed using curettage technique with a sharp curved osteotome followed by a curette. The preparation site is copiously irrigated to remove any interposing cartilage fragments. Next, extensive subchondral drilling in a grid-like pattern is performed followed by "fish-scaling" using a $1/4$-in curved osteotome. It is important that the entire subchondral plate be pulverized and not left intact.

Once this is complete, bone marrow aspirate with or without bone graft can be placed into the fusion site to assist with fusion if deemed necessary.

Following adequate joint preparation, the deformity is corrected. A distal soft tissue procedure/lateral release or medial capsule procedures about the first MTP is performed as needed. The distractor is removed from the medial aspect of the fusion site; however, the distal pin is left in place. Confirmation of the joint position and frontal plane rotation of the first metatarsal and the first IMA can be assessed clinically as well as with fluoroscopy. Next, frontal plane correction can be easily accomplished by

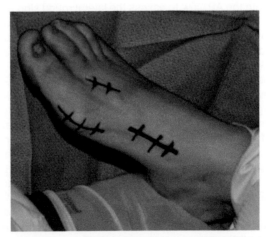

Fig. 1. Incisions are planned over the medial first tarsometatarsal joint, medial eminence, and first interspace.

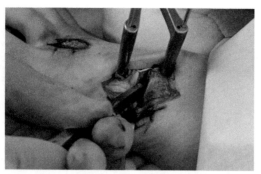

Fig. 2. A pin-based distractor is applied, and the joint is distracted after plantar ligaments are sectioned facilitating joint preparation.

manipulating the distal pin in the first metatarsal so the sesamoids are reduced in anatomic position; this can be done by rotating the distal pin dorsally to the desired position to reduce the valgus deformity by placing the first ray in anatomic alignment (**Fig. 3**A, B).

Via the incision used for lateral release over the first interspace, a large Weber reduction clamp is introduced for IMA correction. The clamp is placed around the neck of the second metatarsal with the other tine directly into the medial aspect of the head of the first metatarsal (**Fig. 3**B, C). The first metatarsal is first derotated using the pin in the metatarsal base; next the clamp is closed to reduce the IMA while dorsiflexing the hallux to plantarflex the metatarsal using the windlass mechanism. Temporary fixation can be applied using guidewires.

The use of cannulated screws allows for accuracy of screw placement. The first guidewire is placed from the central medial base of the first metatarsal, across the first TMT, and into the intermediate cuneiform. This screw creates compression across the TMT joint and imparts enhanced stability of the TMT joint complex. Once the lag screw is inserted, an additional guidewire can be placed from the medial base of the first metatarsal into the base of the second metatarsal. The key to placing this screw is to ensure it is started near the base of the first metatarsal. This screw can be directed

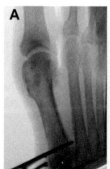
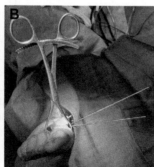
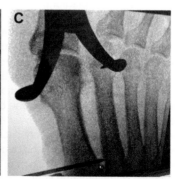

Fig. 3. (*A–C*) (*A*) Wire used for the joint distractor for joint preparation is used to rotate the first metatarsal in the frontal plane. Note the wire in place at the proximal aspect of the first metatarsal. (*B*) Clinical image of the rotation of the distal wire. These wires were parallel when the joint distractor for joint preparation was used. (*C*) A large bone clamp is then used to reduce the IMA. Note the excellent correction of the sesamoid complex.

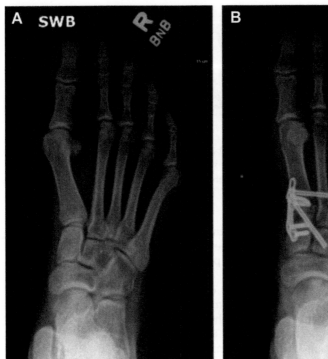
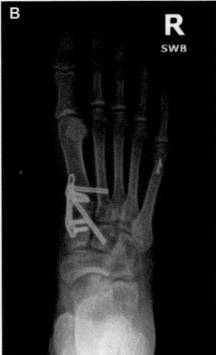

Fig. 4. (*A, B*) Preoperative versus postoperative images demonstrating the addition of supplemental screw from the base of the first metatarsal into the base of the second metatarsal in addition to first metatarsal to intermediate cuneiform.

parallel to the TMTs or even slightly proximal to enter the proximal base of the second metatarsal. The vector pull of this screw trajectory can help close the IMA (**Fig. 4**). The screw should be centered in the second metatarsal and should not drift dorsal or plantar. The first and second metatarsals move independent of each other, and inaccurate placement can create pain or risk of fracture during ambulation. Placing the screw too dorsal/plantar or too distal will likely create stress risers and stress reaction in the second metatarsal bone. Using a partially threaded screw can help close the IMA by compressing the first metatarsal toward the second. A fully threaded screw can be used to help maintain the correction achieved with the standard reduction maneuvers. Headed or headless screws can be used (**Fig. 5**).

Adequate space for fixation at the base of the first metatarsal can be an issue when combining plate and screw fixation, and headless screws can be useful. Burying the head of the screw flush with the bone or placing it slightly plantar to the longitudinal axis allows for plate fixation over and around the screws when necessary. We recommend the use of this additional screw in patients who have a large IMA and/or exhibit high degrees of instability and hypermobility. Preparing the medial base of the second metatarsal can allow for fusion of this area as well and creates a spot weld between the base of the first and second metatarsals. This construct can be particularly helpful in revision cases. Using a screw from the first to second metatarsal bases can be highly effective for bunion correction and intermetatarsal correction. The wounds are closed in layers.

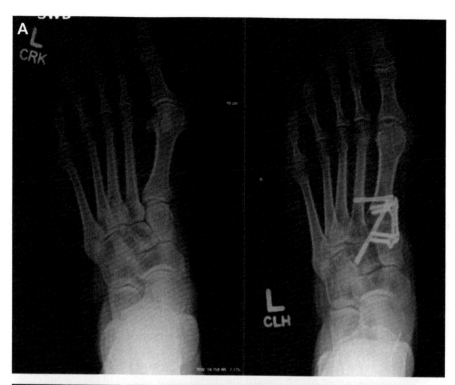

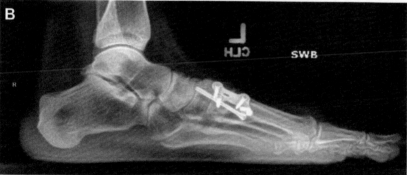

Fig. 5. (*A, B*) AP and lateral radiographs demonstrating addition of a screw from the base of the first metatarsal into the base of the second metatarsal.

ALTERNATIVE TECHNIQUES AND CONSIDERATIONS
The Plantar Lapidus Technique

A 4- to 5-cm incision is made directly over the medial aspect of the first TMT at the level of the superior aspect of the abductor hallucis muscle belly fascia to expose the base of the first metatarsal and medial cuneiform (**Fig. 6**); this is slightly more central medial than our standard technique to allow access to the plantar aspect of the joint.

The joint preparation is performed in the manner described previously using curettage technique. The plantar Lapidus plate is then placed on the inferior surface of the

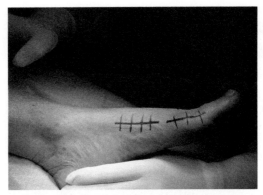

Fig. 6. Medial incisions for access to the first MTP and proximally at the superior aspect of the abductor hallucis muscle belly inferior to the first tarsometatarsal joint.

TMT joint avoiding the insertion of the tibialis anterior tendon. The surgeon must ensure the plate is placed on the cortical surfaces of the medial cuneiform and first metatarsal and it is provisionally fixated to the bone. The locking drill guide is inserted into the plantar distal hole in the plate and the bone is drilled with a 2.5-mm drill bicortically, followed by measurement and insertion of the appropriate-sized screw (**Fig. 7**). Next, the provisional fixation in the distal aspect of the plate is removed and another locking screw is inserted distally. At this time, under fluoroscopic guidance, a drill is passed through the plantar compression hole in the base of the first metatarsal with a 2.5-mm drill and either aimed toward the dorsal lateral aspect of the medial cuneiform or into the intermediate cuneiform (**Fig. 8**A). The first metatarsal is overdrilled with a 4.0-mm drill, followed by measurement and insertion of a 4.0-mm cancellous screw

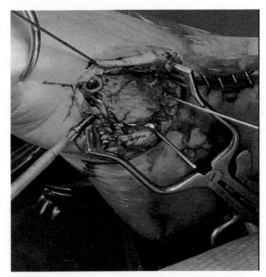

Fig. 7. The plantar Lapidus plate is provisionally fixated to the medial cuneiform, and the distal locking screws are inserted. Note the K-wires at the superior aspect of the fusion site holding the fusion in appropriate position.

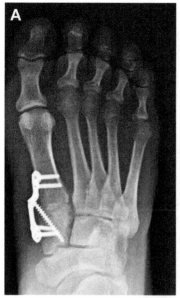
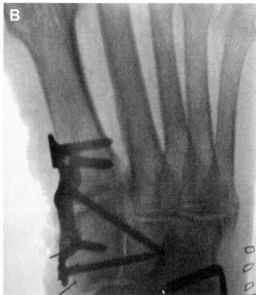

Fig. 8. (*A, B*) The compression screw can be placed into the proximal lateral aspect of the medial cuneiform (*A*) or into the intermediate cuneiform (*B*).

in the compression hole, and before complete tightening of the screw, the provisional K-wire is removed dorsally. Compression of the fusion site is then achieved. At this time the proximal locking screws can be placed into the plate in the same technique as was done distally to complete the construct. To provide additional stabilization an outrigger screw can be placed from the medial cuneiform into the intermediate cuneiform. (**Fig. 8**B). Routine closure is performed, and standard postoperative protocol per surgeon preference is initiated.

3D HALLUX VALGUS CORRECTION

The importance of preoperative sesamoid position, intraoperative reduction, and maintenance of correction through the postoperative course is vital to the 3D hallux valgus correction. The following discussion describes pertinent considerations of the technique to correct hallux valgus in all 3 planes with fixation at the first TMT joint with 2 biplanar plates.

The primary incision is marked out on the dorsum of the first TMT joint immediately adjacent and medial to the extensor hallucis longus. An incision is planned also at the distal aspect of the first webspace to allow access for a lateral collateral ligament release. Next, a crosshatch is placed on the distal aspect of the hallux perpendicular to the nail plate as well as parallel to the nail plate; this allows for easy visualization of deformity correction during and at the completion of the case.

Typically bone marrow aspiration can be taken before tourniquet elevation from the calcaneus as well as procurement of cancellous bone from the lateral aspect of the calcaneus.

Care is taken to release the plantar medial aspect of the first TMT capsule (**Fig. 9**); this will allow for easy rotation in the frontal plane. Next, a sagittal saw is used to plane the saddle-shaped joint into flat surfaces to facilitate rotational correction (**Fig. 10**).

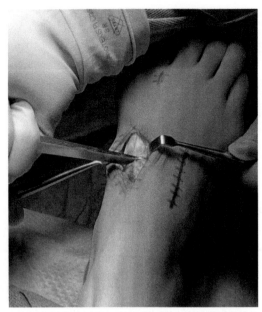

Fig. 9. The incision is carried down to the capsule, and a capsulotomy is performed with an osteotome, focusing on releasing all plantar and medial capsular attachments.

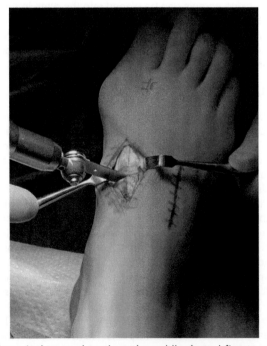

Fig. 10. A sagittal saw is then used to plane the saddle-shaped first tarsometatarsal joint.

Correction of the deformity is obtained with the use of a fulcrum and proprietary compression device that simultaneously corrects all 3 planes of deformity. The goal at this stage is to align the sesamoids and reduce the first IMA on intraoperative AP fluoroscopy. Often there is a substantial medial step-off and visual gap between the base of the first metatarsal and medial cuneiform, which is not a cause for concern. Deformity correction can be seen from the distal hallux before and after correction (**Figs. 11** and **12**).

If the first metatarsal is not parallel to the second metatarsal and the sesamoids are malreduced on fluoroscopy, the reduction jig is repositioned or more aggressive capsular release is needed. Cut guides are used with the angular correction coming primarily from the cuneiform resection. The joint is fenestrated and a compression device is used to bring the bleeding surfaces into contact.

The fixation consists of 2 biplanar plates: one dorsal medial plate is applied with 4 locking screws and a second plate on the medial aspect of the first TMT is applied at 90° to the dorsal plate with 4 locking screws (**Figs. 13** and **14**). No interfragmentary compression screws are used, and this is part of the philosophy of this technique, that rigid compression is not necessary to achieve union. Fluoroscopic guidance is used at this juncture to confirm reduction of sesamoids in the sesamoid axial view as well as AP view.

COMPLICATIONS

When considering the myriad nuances and multiplanar nature of the deformity, a first TMT fusion with triplane realignment is a complex procedure to perform. Adding the component of HAV to an unstable midfoot results in further difficulty in mitigating patient pathology, over the short and long term, in a predictable fashion. Numerous complications can occur and include those ranging from poor technique execution to patient-driven metabolic concerns or noncompliance in the healing phases.

Malreduction in one or all three cardinal planes is a frequently seen complication. In addition, significant shortening of the first metatarsal can occur during debridement of the joint in preparation for fusion, particularly if a saw is used. These complications can

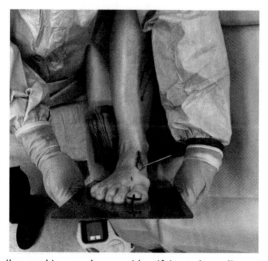

Fig. 11. A distal hallux marking can be seen identifying valgus alignment.

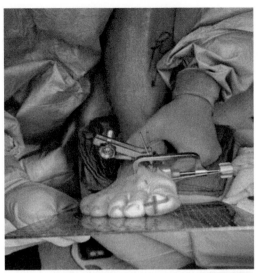

Fig. 12. Deformity correction in the coronal plane can be seen after rotation of the first metatarsal and sesamoid complex.

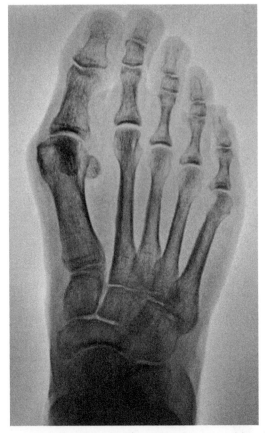

Fig. 13. Preoperative weight-bearing AP demonstrating a positive "round sign" and increased intermetatarsal angle with deviated sesamoid apparatus.

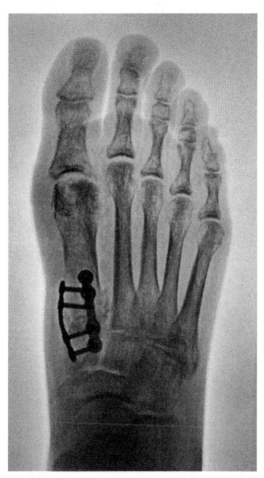

Fig. 14. Three-month radiograph of weight-bearing AP after triplanar hallux valgus correction with biplanar plating.

be mitigated by adhering to strict technical compliance in surgical execution and understanding of intrinsic pathology.

Undercorrection or overcorrection is a potential complication, particularly when one fails to recognize or address the frontal plane component of the deformity. In many cases, a distal metatarsal osteotomy is performed in an inappropriate candidate resulting in recurrence. This technique can present unique challenges when planning and executing a revision with conversion to a Lapidus procedure (**Fig. 15**).

In addition, complications can arise due to inadequate fixation methods or premature weight-bearing protocols in the context of inadequate fixation methods or poor execution of methods described. Any combination therein may create difficulty for the patient and surgeon alike.

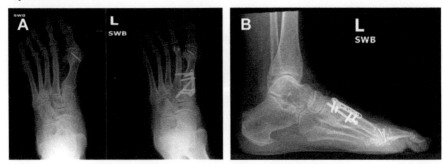

Fig. 15. (*A*) Preoperative AP view with recurrent deformity after distal first metatarsal osteotomy and revision with conversion to first TMT arthrodesis. (*B*). Revision conversion to first TMT arthrodesis with supplemental first to second metatarsal screw and first metatarsal to second cuneiform screw.

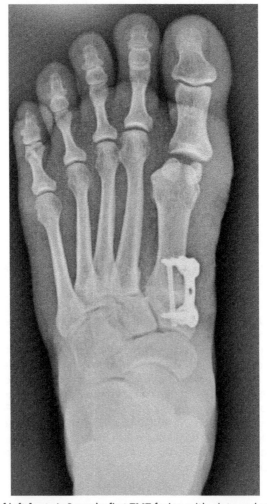

Fig. 16. AP view of left foot s/p 2 weeks first TMT fusion with plate and screw fixation. Note the shortened metatarsal and subluxation of the sesamoids and hallux medially requiring revision.

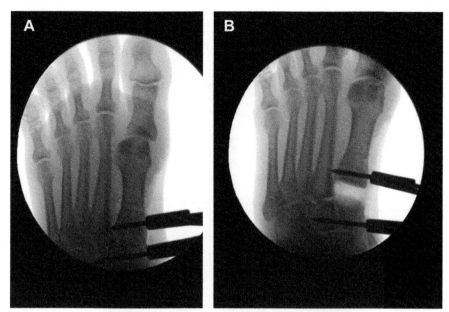

Fig. 17. (*A*, *B*). Intraoperative fluoroscopic AP view of a shortened first metatarsal with application of a pin-to-pin distractor to gain length before graft distraction.

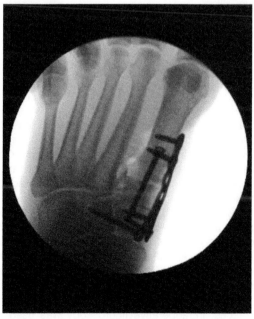

Fig. 18. Final fixation with plate-and-screw construct. Graft application with reduced sesamoid position and parallel first and second metatarsals.

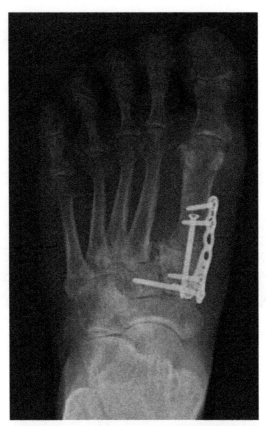

Fig. 19. Six-month weight-bearing radiographs of a revision first tarsometatarsal joint fusion and application of graft distraction with a combination of structural allograft and cancellous autograft.

FIRST TARSOMETATARSAL JOINT REVISION CASE EXAMPLE

A 42-year-old female patient presented 2 weeks status post (s/p) left first TMT joint arthrodesis from an outside institution. She complained of increased pain and concern for position and length of her first metatarsal (**Fig. 16**).

She consented for a revision first TMT fusion with possible bone grafting. Intraoperatively, via the same incisional approach, hardware was stable and removed without incident. There were no signs of infection. The joint was prepared for fusion via curettage technique to maintain length; 5 cc of autogenous cancellous bone was procured from the lateral calcaneus with a dowel reamer as well as 5 cc of bone marrow aspirate. A pin-to-pin spreader was used to distract the joint. Adequate length was obtained on Fluoroscan, and clinical appearance of the nail plate was parallel to the weight-bearing surface of the foot (**Fig. 17**). The gap was measured to be 12 mm, and an iliac crest allograft was fashioned on the back table to the appropriate size and shape. The graft was soaked in the aspirate for 5 minutes, and our cancellous bone was packed in between the first and second metatarsal bases as well as any adjacent open interfaces. Intraoperative fluoroscopy was used to determine final reduction of the deformity. The goal was reduction of the sesamoid apparatus and

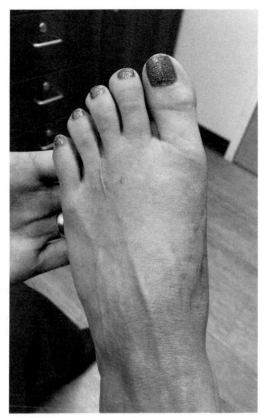

Fig. 20. Clinical appearance of a revision first tarsometatarsal joint fusion. Note hallux nail plate parallel to the weight-bearing surface of the foot.

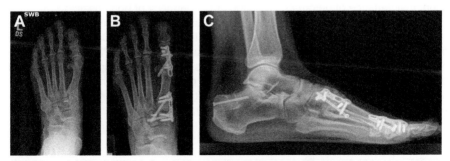

Fig. 21. (*A*) AP radiograph demonstrating failed Lapidus with chronic nonunion and shortening of the first ray. (*B, C*) Revision Lapidus with distraction arthrodesis using structural graft from the calcaneus. Note restoration of first ray length with solid union and fixation of allograft with complete incorporation at harvest site.

appropriate reduction of the lateral round sign on the first metatarsal head as well as restoration of the appropriate metatarsal length parabola. Fixation was applied with a noncompressive, fully threaded 3.5-mm cortical screw from distal to proximal and a medial neutralization plate (**Fig. 18**). Closure was performed in standard fashion, and a compressive dressing and splint were used. The patient was non-weight-bearing for 8 weeks. Progressive weight-bearing in a fracture boot was started at 8 weeks followed by physical therapy.

Patient presented at 6-month follow-up pain free, weight-bearing in normal supportive shoe gear with solid union and excellent alignment (**Figs. 19** and **20**).

REVISION FIRST TARSOMETATARSAL JOINT FUSION CASE 2

A failed Lapidus can create a difficult situation for the surgeon and patient. In the case of a failed arthrodesis of the first TMT joint, there can be significant shortening along with continued malalignment. In this case, the surgeon needs to consider the best way to gain length and allow for joint healing. A structural calcaneal autograft can be obtained from the posterior superior body of the calcaneus. A vertical incision is placed along the lateral body of the calcaneus just anterior to the Achilles tendon. A saw is used to create an osteotomy to the length needed in the posterior/superior/lateral body of the calcaneus. An osteotome is used to free the graft from the calcaneus. The bone void is filled with allograft bone and fixated with a single screw. When preparing the first TMT joint, any nonviable bone should be resected and a good bleeding base should be created. Biologics can be used. The structural autograft should be placed in the joint using a distractor and one should ensure to get the angular correction desired. Including the intermediate cuneiform in the construct will create added stability (**Fig. 21**).

POSTOPERATIVE PROTOCOL

Patients are placed into a short leg non weight bearing splint or cast during the first two postoperative weeks. At week 2, the sutures are removed and the patient is transitioned into a tall CAM Boot in an effort to allow for early weight-bearing while mitigating cantilever forces through the fusion site and continuing to shield the fusion mass. Range of motion exercises also begin at the second week, including dorsiflexion and plantarflexion at the first MTP. Range of motion can also begin at the ankle joint; however, weight bearing as tolerated should remain in the Cam Boot.

Serial radiographs are obtained at each postoperative visit to ensure stability of fixation, maintenance of deformity reduction, and adequacy of bone healing.

At the 6-week postoperative interval, as long as the radiographic examination indicates stability of fusion, the patient can be transitioned out of the Cam Boot gradually over a period of days into a sports-type brace and regular shoes. Activities at the 6-week interval can include nonballistic activities, such as walking, swimming, and biking. The patient will also be encouraged to perform formal physical therapy for range of motion, balance, strengthening, and gait pattern training. More ballistic-type activity can progress based on patient tolerance.

CLINICS CARE POINTS

- Joint curettage preparation preserves length of the first ray
- Adequate soft tissue release at the TMT joint and MTP joint level will allow for frontal plane deformity correction. Release of the metatarsal sesamoid ligament is key to the reduction.

- A distraction pin from a pin-based distractor in the medial first metatarsal can be used as a joystick to derotate the metatarsal out of valgus
- Clamp placement around the first metatarsal head and second metatarsal neck will close the IMA after derotating in the frontal plane. The clamp is placed before medial eminence resection to avoid bone collapse
- Placement of the cross screw to the intermediate cuneiform will add stability to the construct
- Placement of a screw from the first metatarsal base to the second metatarsal base can assist in IMA closure and maintain deformity correction
- Dorsiflexion of the hallux using the windlass mechanism prevents first ray elevation while compressing the Weber clamp to reduce the IMA.
- Place the medial screw from the first metatarsal base to intermediate cuneiform inferior enough to allow placement of the locking plate without interference. An alternative is to countersink the screw head to allow it to be placed flush with the bone.
- Screw threads for the first metatarsal to intermediate cuneiform should all be within the intermediate cuneiform because threads bridging the intercuneiform joint can result in subtle distraction resulting in increase of the IMA.
- Positioning the fluoroscopy unit on the same side of the operative limb. The scrub technician should be situated on the opposite side of the bed; this allows for appropriate imaging and efficiency in the operating room.

DISCLOSURE

M.D., Dujela DePuy Synthes; T. Langan, Medline; J. Cottom, Arthrex; W.T. DeCarbo, Treace Medical; J.E. McAlister, Treace Medical; C.F. Hyer, Wright Medical.

REFERENCES

1. Lapidus PW. The operative correction of the metatarsus varus primus in hallux valgus. Surg Gynecol Obstet 1934;58:183, 1-7.
2. Albrecht GH. The pathology and treatment of hallux valgus. Russ Vrach 1911;10: 14. Russian.
3. Langan TM, Brandão RA, Goss DA Jr, et al. Arthrodesis of the first tarsometatarsal joint for correction of hallux abductovalgus: technique guide and tips. Foot Ankle Surg Tech Rep Cases 2021;1(2):100008.
4. Langan TM, Greschner JM, Brandão RA, et al. Maintenance of correction of the modified lapidus procedure with a first metatarsal to intermediate cuneiform cross-screw technique. Foot Ankle Int 2020;41(4):428–36.
5. Coughlin MJ. Instructional course lectures, the American Academy of Orthopaedic Surgeons-Hallux Valgus. J Bone Joint Surg Am 1996;78(6):932–66.
6. Coughlin MJ, Jones CP. Hallux valgus and first ray mobility: a prospective study. J Bone Joint Surg AM 2007;89(9):1887–98.
7. Scanton PE, Rutkowski R. Anatomic variations in the first ray: Part I. Anatomic aspects related to bunion surgery. Clin Orthop Relat Res 1980;151:244–55.
8. Dayton P, Feilmeier M, Hirschi J, et al. Observed changes in radiographic measurement of the first ray after frontal plane rotation of the first metatarsal in a Cadaveric Foot Model. J Foot Ankle Surg 2014;53(3):274–8.
9. Welck MJ, Al-Khudairi N. Imaging of hallux valgus: how to approach the deformity. Foot Ankle Clin 2018;23(2):183–92.

10. Shibuya N, Roukis TS, Jupiter DC. Mobility of the first ray in patients with or without hallux valgus deformity: systematic review and meta-analysis. J Foot Ankle Surg 2017;56(5):1070–5.

11. King DM, Toolan BC. Associated deformities and hypermobility in hallux valgus: an investigation with weightbearing radiographs. Foot Ankle Int 2004;25(4): 251–5.

12. Barouk LS. The effect of gastrocnemius tightness on the pathogenesis of juvenile hallux valgus: a Preliminary Study. Foot Ankle Clin 2014;19(4):807–22.

13. Okuda R, Kinoshita M, Yasuda T, et al. The shape of the lateral edge of the first metatarsal head as a risk factor for recurrence of hallux valgus. J Bone Joint Surg AM 2007;89(10):2163–72.

14. Coughlin MJ, Saltzman CL, Nunley JA. Angular measurements in the evaluation of hallux valgus deformities: a report of the ad hoc committee of the American Orthopaedic Foot & Ankle Society on angular measurements. Foot Ankle Int 2002; 23(1):68–74.

15. Coughlin MJ, Freund E. Roger A Mann Award: the reliability of angular measurements in hallux valgus deformities. Foot Ankle Int 2001;22(5):369–79.

16. Lee KM, Ahn S, Chung CY, et al. Reliability and relationship of radiographic measurements in hallux valgus. Clin Orthop Relat Res 2012;470(9):2613–21.

17. Dayton P, Feilmeier M, Kauwe M, et al. Observed changes in radiographic measurements of the first ray after frontal and transverse plane rotation of the hallux: does the hallux drive the metatarsal in a bunion deformity? J Foot Ankle Surg 2014;53(5):584–7.

18. Dayton P, Feilmeier M. Comparison of tibial sesamoid position on anteroposterior and axial radiographs before and after triplane tarsal metatarsal joint arthrodesis. J Foot Ankle Surg 2017;56(5):1041–6.

19. Dayton P, Feilmeier M, Kauwe M, et al. Relationship of frontal plane rotation of first metatarsal to proximal articular set angle and hallux alignment in patients undergoing tarsometatarsal arthrodesis for hallux abducto valgus: a case series and critical review of the literature. J Foot Ankle Surg 2013;52(3):348–54.

20. Hardy RH, Clapham JCR. Observations on hallux valgus: based on a controlled series. J Bone Joint Surg Br 1951;33-B(3):376–91.

21. Okuda R, Kinoshita M, Yasuda T, et al. Postoperative incomplete reduction of the sesamoids as a risk factor for recurrence of hallux valgus. J Bone Joint Surg Am 2009;91(7):1637–45.

22. Talbot KD, Saltman CL. Assessing sesamoid subluxation: how good is the AP radiograph? Foot Ankle Int 1998;19(8):547–54.

23. Pentikainen I, Ojala R, Ohtonen P, et al. Preoperative radiogical factors correlated to long-term recurrence of hallux valgus following distal chevron osteotomy. Foot Ankle Int 2014;35:1262–7.

24. Hatch DJ, Santrock RD, Smith B, et al. Triplane hallux abducto valgus classification. J Foot Ankle Surg 2018;57:972–81.

Soft Tissue Reconstruction and Osteotomies for Pes Planovalgus Correction

Jason George DeVries, DPM[a],*, William T. DeCarbo, DPM[b,1],
Ryan T. Scott, DPM[c], Brad Bussewitz, DPM[d],
Mitchell Thompson, DPM, AACFAS[e,2], Christopher F. Hyer, DPM, MS[f,g]

KEYWORDS

- Posterior tibialis tendon dysfunction (PTTD) • Calcaneal osteotomy
- Adult-acquired flatfoot • Spring ligament • Cotton osteotomy

KEY POINTS

- The authors discuss the reconstructive options for repair of the collapsed pes planovalgus foot.
- Joint sparing surgery requires a comprehensive approach to the entire deformity, we care to address the mechanical, bony, and soft tissue concerns.
- The authors discuss the rational for procedure choice, as well as techniques and pearls for the surgical procedures.

INTRODUCTION

Pes planovalgus (PPV), adult-acquired flatfoot deformity (AAFD), or posterior tibialis tendon dysfunction (PTTD) is a wide ranging and complicated topic. It encompasses a wide range of severity, apices, staging, as well as bony and soft tissue components. Significant literature review has focused on various treatment modalities, with no "one

[a] Board Certified, Foot & Ankle Reconstructive Surgery, Orthopedics & Sports Medicine – BayCare Clinic, 1111 Bayshore Dr, Manitowoc, WI 54220, USA; [b] Board Certified, Foot & Ankle Reconstructive Surgery, St. Clair Orthopedic Associates, Pittsburgh, PA 15243, USA; [c] Board Certified, Foot & Ankle Reconstructive Surgery, The CORE Institute Foot and Ankle Reconstruction Fellowship, The CORE Institute, 9321 West Thomas Road, Suite 205, Phoenix, AZ 85037, USA; [d] Board Certified, Foot & Ankle Reconstructive Surgery, Steindler Orthopedic Clinic, 2751 Northgate Drive, Iowa City, IA 52245, USA; [e] Orthopedic Foot and Ankle Center, Worthington, OH, USA; [f] Board Certified, Foot & Ankle Reconstructive Surgery, Orthopedic Foot & Ankle Center, Columbus, OH, USA; [g] Orthopedic Foot & Ankle Center, 350 West Wilson Bridge Road, Suite 200, Worthington, OH 43085, USA
[1] Present address: 1768 Sapphire Court, Pittsburgh, PA 15241.
[2] Present address: 3255 McKinley Avenue, Apartment 427, Columbus, OH 43204.
* Corresponding author.
E-mail address: jdevries@baycare.net

Clin Podiatr Med Surg 39 (2022) 207–231
https://doi.org/10.1016/j.cpm.2021.11.010
0891-8422/22/© 2021 Elsevier Inc. All rights reserved.

size fits all" approach being possible for adequate correction. The authors will present a sampling of the most common and useful surgical procedures for use in this condition, including indications and technique.

The spectrum of deformity has long been recognized and classified. In 1989, Johnson and Strom classified the foot deformity into 3 stages.[1] Stage 1 is present when there is pain present at the medial foot and ankle along the posterior tibialis tendon (PTT), but without the associated deformity and functional deficit. Stage 2 involves pain along the medial ankle, but now encompasses a mobile but deformed foot. This is characterized by heel valgus, forefoot abduction, and a general loss of the medial longitudinal arch of the foot. Within this stage, there are subgroups breaking this into mild cases with limited functional loss, and more severe (but still reducible) cases with functional loss, particularly the loss of the single heel rise. Stage 3 represents deformity that is isolated to the foot but is incompletely reducible and may have significant hindfoot arthritis and adaptive changes of the bone structure. In 1996, Myerson added a stage 4, and this involved ankle deformity for which the eccentric forces of the valgus and abducted foot caused stress and eventual incompetence of the deltoid ligament of the medial ankle.[2] Stage 1 is typically treated nonoperatively, stage 3 typically requires hindfoot realignment arthrodesis, and stage 4 requires additional surgical work at the ankle. Stage 2 is the most controversial and wide-ranging stage and can be treated with joint preserving soft tissue rebalancing and osteotomy realignment of the hindfoot and forefoot.[3] This is the focus of the present chapter.

While conservative measures for earlier stages of AAFD have evidence of success,[4] if these measures fail, surgical options are considered. In the case of a flexible deformity and a lack of arthritic changes, joint sparing surgery is preferred. This encompasses a host of different soft tissue rebalancing procedures and bony realignment osteotomies. Deciphering the appropriate indications for specific procedures is paramount to successful outcomes. In addition, technical soundness and efficiency are critical as often there are many procedures that need to be performed in the same setting. The ability to perform multiple operations in a single surgical setting will help the patient by going through only one surgical episode and doing this quickly will decrease the potential for wound complications, tourniquet issues, and infection. The authors will outline their indications as well as technique and pearls for joint sparing soft tissue and bony procedures.

SOFT TISSUE RECONSTRUCTION
Kidner – When?

In 1929, Kidner proposed a treatment for painful accessory navicular tuberosity, or os tibiale externum (OTE). The report suggested that the accessory bone affected the insertion of the PTT and put it at a biomechanical disadvantage. The Kidner procedure proposed removing the accessory bone and rerouting the tendon to the plantar surface of the navicular tuberosity. This sought to restore the biomechanical pull and correct a weak longitudinal arch.[5]

While the results of the Kidner procedure are generally favorable, it has been shown to not be able to radiographically correct the medial longitudinal arch. A study in 2004 by Kopp and Marcus demonstrated that while all the 13 patients were satisfied with the procedure, none of them had any significant change in arch alignment.[6] Similarly, a report in 1995 by Prichasuk and Sinphurmsukskul showed good results in pain and fatigue in 27 out of 28 patients (96%). However, only 3 out of 25 patients (12%) had any improvement in the medial arch.[7] In addition to these findings, several papers have evaluated the findings in revision surgery for patients after a Kidner procedure. In 2017, Choi and Lee looked at 9 patients requiring revision surgery and found that

78% had a planovalgus deformity,[8] and in 2020, Kim and colleagues[9] found that 20 out of 21 patients (95%) had a heel valgus alignment. There are some controversies as to whether the valgus was present before surgery, or developed after the operation, but there seems to be a connection.

When considering the Kidner procedure in the face of a flatfoot deformity, it should never be performed in isolation. By simply excising the accessory bone and advancing the tendon, without the consideration and correction of the foot deformity, the patient is at significantly increased risk of failure. Even if the primary concern is the painful OTE, the potential flatfoot must be addressed.

Indications

There are however some indications for the Kidner procedure when the main concern is the AAFD. Certainly a Kidner procedure is indicated in the presence of a large, symptomatic OTE (**Fig. 1**). Even in this case, at least a medial calcaneal displacement osteotomy should be performed. In a flat foot, it should be considered when there is a concomitant OTE, as this will need to be removed to retension and realign the pull of the PTT. Also, it can be considered even in a modified fashion in the face of a preoperative MRI that shows no damage or tearing to the PTT. Again, after hindfoot alignment, the Kidner procedure can be performed even without a true accessory bone simply to tighten up the PTT. Finally, consideration for a Kidner procedure should be given in a pediatric population. These patients may have more ability to adapt after tendon advancement and it may not be necessary to transfer the flexor digitorum longus (FDL).

Technique

An incision is made over the course of the PTT insertion and is carried distal to the navicular tuberosity. Carry this to the tendon sheath which is opened. The main

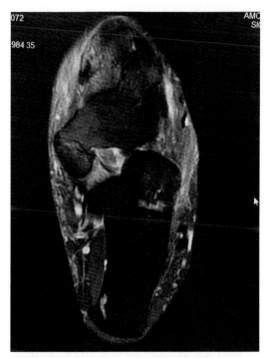

Fig. 1. T2 MRI image showing a large os tibiale externum (OTE) with associated bone marrow edema. This is an indication of a Kidner procedure.

attachment of the PTT is released, while the plantar and recurrent attachments may be left intact. In cases of a true accessory bone, this is excised. Then, the medial aspect of the navicular tuberosity is resected (**Fig. 2**). Care is taken to avoid the disruption of the talonavicular or naviculocuneiform joints and can be started with osteotome or sagittal saw. The reattachment site of the PTT is then determined, and an anchor is placed. This is central from anterior to posterior and angled from plantar-medial to dorsal-lateral. The punch is placed visually, but then confirmed radiographically (**Fig. 3**). The area can then be tapped and the anchor placed. The attached sutures for the 5.5 mm anchor are used to reattach the tendon to the navicular bone at the raw bone surface. Place one suture in a running nonlocking suture technique proximal and distal within the tendon. A second suture then has both ends of the suture placed from deep to superficial through the PTT, with care taken to incorporate the previous running suture (**Fig. 4**). First, the running suture is tied down, with the knot buried in the reattachment site. Then the horizontal type of suture is tied down to pull the entire attachment in a broad footprint. The periphery of the attachment is then tied down with 0 Vicryl.

Pearls

- Not only the OTE but also the medial navicular tuberosity should be removed to provide a good bony surface for tendon attachment and to realign the biomechanical pull.
- While the main attachment of the PTT is detached, the plantar and recurrent aspects of the PTT may be left in place.
- Use an anchor with multiple sutures attached to make repair with a running and horizontal repair easier.

Posterior Tibialis Tendon Repair Versus Resection, Flexor Digitorum Longus Transfer

The posterior tibial tendon is a dynamic stabilizer of the medial arch and the most powerful inverter of the foot.[10,11] Pathology such as the longitudinal rupture or dysfunction of the tendon often leads to pain in the medial arch. If conservative treatment fails patients are often faced with the option to surgically reconstruct the deformity. Most posterior tibial tendon dysfunction surgery involves addressing the

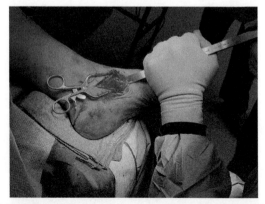

Fig. 2. Removal of the OTE and prominent medial navicular tuberosity. This is usually started with an osteotome to avoid skin damage, and then may be finished with a sagittal saw. Avoid resecting into the naviculocuneiform (NC) or talonavicular (TN) joints.

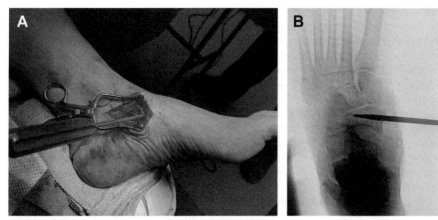

Fig. 3. (*A*) Punch for the anchor is placed plantar-medially to reattach the posterior tibialis tendon (PTT). (*B*) Intraoperative fluoroscopy confirms placement avoids damage to the NC and TN joints.

pathologic posterior tibial tendon in some way. The options with regards to how to handle the posterior tibial tendon include a direct repair, resection of the tendon, transfer of the adjacent FDL tendon or a combination of the aforementioned. One of the challenges with repair of the posterior tibial tendon is the adjacent tendon (FDL), which is most commonly transferred to augment or take the place of the PTT, is two times smaller than the PT tendon.[12] This presents a challenge to replace a muscle/tendon complex of this size and strength. Any repair, resection, or replacement of the posterior tibial tendon is usually reserved for Johnson and Strom stage 1 or 2 A/B as the foot is still flexible. The surgical goals are to restore the posterior tibial tendon function and correct the deformity. It is often necessary to implement bone procedures in addition to the medial soft tissue repair to protect the medial repair over time.[13,14] When it comes to whether to keep the posterior tibial tendon or resect it 2 trains of thought persist. One is the tendon is a pain generator and must be removed, the other is the PT tendon is stronger than the potential muscle/tendons being transferred so the PT tendon must be preserved.[15]

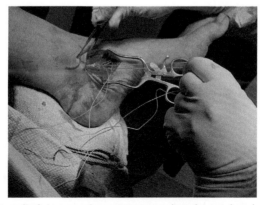

Fig. 4. The first suture limb is a running suture to anchor the tendon deep, and the second suture is a horizontal suture encompassing the running suture.

Indications

The decision to preserve the posterior tibial tendon is not only because it is the strongest of the medial foot structures but it also balances against the peroneal longus and brevis tendon maintaining an appropriate balance of the foot.[15] Primary repair of the posterior tibial tendon with debridement alone should be reserved for patients without deformity.[16] Gould[17] recommended primary repair in patients with acute mid-substance ruptures stating longitudinal ruptures with minimal lengthening and weakness can be debulked and tubularized. With primary repair and deformity of the hindfoot and midfoot concomitant bone procedures are recommended. Realignment of the hindfoot decreases the mechanical advantage of the peroneal brevis tendon and decreases the strain on the PT tendon by 51%.[9] For this reason, it is recommended and common practice to protect the medial soft tissue repair with hindfoot bone procedures.

The argument has been made to resect the diseased PT tendon for multiple reasons. The pathologic tendon is hypertrophied with the loss of normal appearance and function. The degenerated tendinosis is made up of disorganized collagen.[18–20] It has also been stated that if the hypertrophied tendon is not resected then the addition of a tendon transfer adds too much bulk to the medial arch.[15] Rosenfeld and colleagues[21] reported that PT excision with FDL transfer resulted in a more functional performance of the foot. They noted the FDL muscle hypertrophied as much as 44% and the PT muscle underwent atrophy by 23%. In the same study, the FDL muscle only hypertrophied by 11% with the PT tendon retained. The FDL tendon adapts to the force needed after the PT tendon was excised. They reported outcomes for PTTD reconstruction in patients that had the PT tendon excised with the transfer of the FDL to the navicular with the addition of a medial displacement calcaneal osteotomy.

Regarding the transfer of the FDL tendon with the preservation of the posterior tibial tendon, the goal is to counteract the peroneal brevis tendon. The combination of the FDL transfer with the remaining strength of the PT tendon is said to be adequate to support the medial arch.[22] The FDL tendon is in the same area of the PT tendon and can be accessed through the same incision, the FDL does not cross the neurovascular bundle and it is in the same phase of gait with similar excursion as the PT tendon.[23] Another positive is the distal function can be preserved when resection of the FDL is made proximal to the Knot of Henry. There are several ways to fixate the transferred tendon including side to side anastomosis, anchors into the medial navicular, or the use of a bone tunnel through the navicular attaching the FDL back to itself or using interference screws.

Technique

A medial incision is made approximately 6 to 8 cm from the tip of the medial malleolus to 1 cm distal to the navicular tubercle along the course of the PT tendon. Dissection is carried into the PT tendon sheath and the PT tendon is identified and the medial and inferior insertion to the navicular is released. At this time, the decision to debride and repair or excise the tendon can be made. If the PT tendon is preserved it is retracted superiorly and dissection is continued into the FDL tendon sheath which is directly behind and slightly inferior to whereby the PT tendon courses (**Fig. 5**). The FDL tendon is released at the Knot of Henry and with the ankle and lesser digits in maximum plantarflexion, the tendon is cut. A tendon passing stitch is made through the distal end and the FDL is retracted out of the incision area. If a bone tunnel technique is used a bone tunnel through the navicular from inferior to superior is made with an appropriate sized drill bit (**Fig. 6**). A tendon passer is used to transfer the FDL through the bone tunnel from inferior to superior (**Fig. 7**). With the foot held in slight inversion

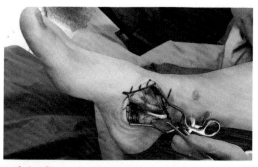

Fig. 5. Identification of the flexor digitorum longus (FDL) deep and inferior to the PTT.

the FDL tendon is sutured onto itself. An interference screw can also be used either for primary or secondary fixation. The PT tendon is then advanced and repair back to the navicular and the FDL and PT tendon are reinforced with side-to-side anastomosis (**Fig. 8**).

Pearls

- Little evidence to support resection of the PT tendon versus maintaining it.
- If the PT tendon is not significantly degenerated it is recommended to leave it.
- FDL tendon is a common and best choice for transfer to augment a pathologic PT tendon.

Spring Ligament Repair

Recently, spring ligament pathology has gained some popularity. Reviewing the literature shows that spring ligament repair was described as early as 1992.[24,25]

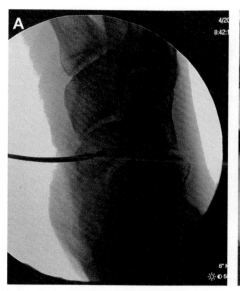
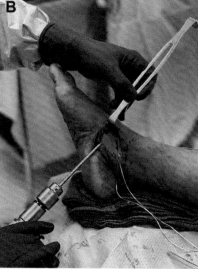

Fig. 6. (*A*) Guidewire placement to confirm central location in the navicular to allow for a bone tunnel. (*B*) Drill over the guidewire from plantar to dorsal to make the tunnel.

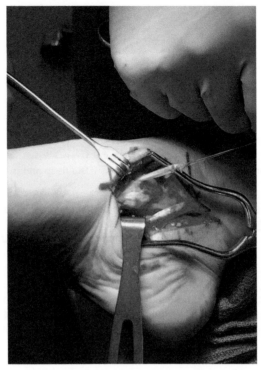

Fig. 7. The FDL is passed from the plantar to dorsal through the navicular bone tunnel and tensioned.

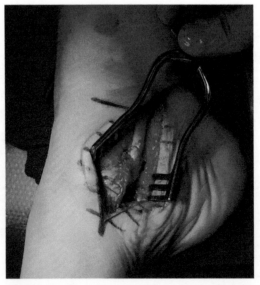

Fig. 8. Final repair with FDL transfer and side-to-side anastomosis of the viable aspect of the PTT after adequate debridement.

Deland[25] indicates that the spring ligament complex is the major stabilizer of the arch during midstance and that the posterior tibial tendon is incapable of fully accommodating for its insufficiency, suggesting that the spring ligament complex should be evaluated and, if indicated, repaired in flatfoot reconstruction. If not treated, consequences such as acquired flatfoot deformity and loss of correction of treated flatfoot may result.[26] Isolated spring ligament repair in the face of posterior tibial tendon dysfunction is not typically recommended, and other bony procedures need to be undertaken.[27]

Different materials have been described in the augmentation for spring ligament repair. Originally described as a simple repair,[28] reconstruction of the spring ligament using either hamstring allograft or synthetic ligament augmentation provided significant improvements in radiological alignment; however, superior patient-reported outcomes were found in the synthetic ligament augmentation group.[29] Suture tape system reconstruction showed an increased number of patients with single leg stance and better correction of forefoot abduction.[30]

Indications

Spring ligament repair is considered in AAFD with peri-talar subluxation and laxity of the posterior tibial tendon, spring ligament tear, and laxity of the spring ligament following osseous correction. It is typically performed in conjunction with a posterior tibial tendon debridement and repair with an FDL tendon transfer. The addition of the spring ligament repair will further strengthen the medial soft tissue construct and further reduce the risk of reoccurrence. The use of MRI will help to identify the integrity of the spring ligament and the medial soft tissue structures. On weight-bearing radiographs the talar head will be declinated, indicated by a talonavicular joint fault.

Technique

Incision is following the posterior tibial tendon repair incision. Dissection is then taken through the posterior tibial tendon sheath, exposing the posterior tibial tendon. Dissection is immediately taken inferior and slightly posterior. The FDL is then exposed and retracted superior. Inspection of the spring ligament is then performed in its entirety.

The demonstrated reconstruction includes the use of a synthetic augmentation/ suture tape construct. The medial aspect of the subtalar joint is identified with a range of motion. The sustentaculum is identified and cleared of any soft tissue adhesions. A guidewire is placed in the central aspect of the sustentaculum tali and driven in a lateral and slightly plantar fashion. Lateral and calcaneal axial views are obtained to ensure the placement of the guidewire to avoid the floor of the sinus tarsi (**Fig. 9**). The drill is then used to create a bone tunnel. The synthetic augmentation/suture tape is then secured into the sustentaculum tali via a blind hole approach leaving a superior and inferior limb (**Fig. 10**). A bone tunnel is then created in the medial pole of the navicular. This is typically performed in conjunction with the FDL tendon transfer. The superior limb is then transferred underneath the posterior tibial tendon against the medial aspect of the talus. The limbs of the augmentation are then passed from superior to inferior, and inferior to superior through the osseous tunnel in the navicular. This forms a triangular appearance with the apex at the sustentaculum. With the foot in neutral and the talonavicular joint reduced the augmentation and FDL are fixated with a tenodesis anchor. This augmentation stabilizes the medial talonavicular joint by adding a medial and plantar endpoint (**Fig. 11**).

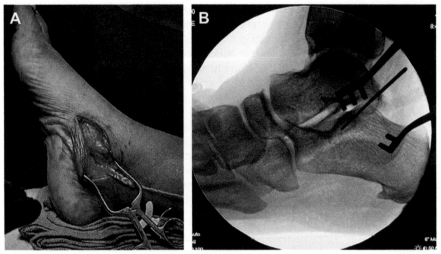

Fig. 9. (*A*) Identification of the sustentaculum tali deep and inferior to the FDL tendon. (*B*) Fluoroscopic confirmation of the guidewire in the sustentaculum tali for blind tunnel placement to anchor to synthetic spring ligament.

Pearls

- When performing the spring ligament repair in conjunction with the FDL tendon transfer up half-size on the reamer when creating the navicular osseous tunnel. The synthetic augmentation/suture tape will add extra volume to the transfer.
- Pull the superior to inferior limb before the FDL and the inferior limb into the bone tunnel.
- Transfer the FDL tendon and the inferior limb simultaneous.

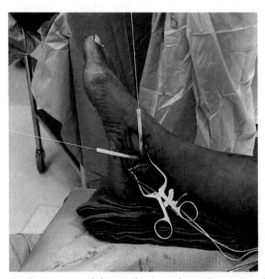

Fig. 10. Superior and inferior arms of the synthetic graft used to repair the spring ligament after anchoring into the sustentaculum tali.

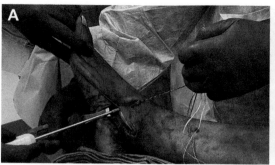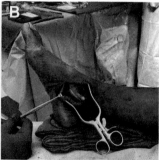

Fig. 11. (*A*) With the synthetic graft tensioned and the FDL tendon through the osseous tunnel in the navicular, an interference screw is placed. (*B*) Final construct demonstrates the final appearance of the FDL transfer with spring ligament reconstruction.

- Maintain tension on the superior to inferior limb during insertion of the plantar to dorsal interference screw.

OSTEOTOMIES
Medial Displacement Calcaneal Osteotomy

One of the most powerful procedures of a flat foot reconstruction is the medial displacement calcaneal osteotomy (MDCO). The medial displacement calcaneal osteotomy was originally popularized by Koutsogiannis in 1971.[31] This medial slide of the posterior tuberosity of the calcaneus focuses on the frontal plane dominant flatfoot deformity. It works by medializing the ground reactive forces and pull of the Achilles tendon.[32,33]

Indications

The medial slide is often used in conjunction with repair of the PTT and flexor digitorum tendon transfer.[12,34] As stated, it is used in the frontal plane dominant flatfoot, and when the heel valgus is the prime deformity. It can be used in conjunction with a lateral column lengthening (LCL). When compared with an LCL, it has been shown to have better 1st ray plantarflexion and varus position but does have a higher rate of reoperation.[35,36]

Technique

The incision is created obliquely at the lateral calcaneus and created in line with the expected osteotomy. The incision is deepened sharply to the lateral wall of the calcaneus. A Cobb or key elevator is used to establish a clear visual field of the osteotomy site. A lateral image can be taken to verify osteotomy location and electrocautery can be used to mark the osteotomy.

A deep soft tissue retractor is placed and Hohmann retractors can be used at both ends of the osteotomy to protect soft tissue from saw excursion. The cut is created perpendicular to the lateral wall of the calcaneus and to the long axis of the tuber. The medial wall of the calcaneus will be felt with the saw blade near completion of the cut and a half-inch straight osteotome is used to complete the cut to protect the nearby medial neurovascular structures.

A lamina spreader is now placed within the bone cut and used to open the osteotomy and stretch the medial soft tissue in preparation for the translation (**Fig. 12**). Cannulated wires can be advanced through the posterior calcaneus with the lamina

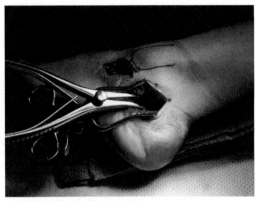

Fig. 12. Lamina spreader is placed into the calcaneal osteotomy and spread. This will help mobilize the posterior tuber and stretch the medial structures.

spreader in place to visualize the wire position as the wires enter the osteotomy (**Fig. 13**). With the lamina spreader now removed, the calcaneus can be slid straight medially up to 1 cm, depending on the correction desired. Avoid translating the calcaneus dorsally.

Two cannulated 4.5mm–6.5 mm partially threaded screws (**Fig. 14**), or a specialized step plate and screws or staple can be used (**Fig. 15**). The calcaneal axial view is useful to visualize hardware position and translation. The screws are advanced as far as the anterior cortex in a normal fashion. Avoid leaving the screw heads proud, as this can be the source of irritation. The prominent lateral edge of the calcaneal wall at the step-off can now be beveled with a rongeur or impacted flush with a tamp.

Pearls

- A sterile bump under the heel makes it efficient to float the heel as needed for mobilization and screw insertion.
- Care must be taken to avoid the sural nerve during dissection.
- After translation of the posterior tuber, with one hand the toes can be dorsiflexed to engage the windlass mechanism and the medialized tuber will remain stable.

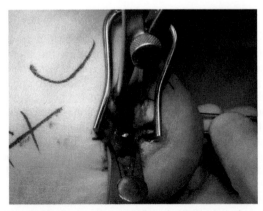

Fig. 13. Guidewires for the fixation screws are placed percutaneously in the posterior tuber and visualized in the osteotomy to confirm proper placement.

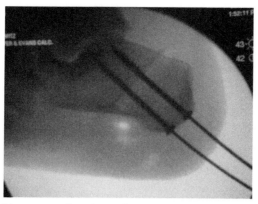

Fig. 14. Screws are driven across the calcaneal osteotomy site. Care is taken to make sure the threads cross the osteotomy site and the heads are not proud.

Evans Calcaneal Osteotomy

The LCL was first described by Dillwyn Evans in 1975 for the correction of a calcaneo-valgus foot.[37] It consists of an osteotomy in the anterior process of the calcaneus that is lengthened and a graft is placed. Comparison of allograft and autograft bone wedges favors allograft placement.[38,39] There was some concern on the effect on the calcaneocuboid pressure and the potential for developing arthritis. However, this was noted in a normally aligned cadaveric specimen and did not seem to be a concern in a flatfoot model.[40,41]

Indications
The LCL has been indicated in a transverse plane dominant flatfoot deformity (**Fig. 16**). It can provide for triplane correction of the collapsed foot. It does so with tensioning of the plantar ligaments and by locking of the midtarsal joint. When compared with the medial displacement calcaneal osteotomy, the LCL provides better heel inversion. It also provides greater initial and maintained correction but does have a higher potential for nonunion and adjacent joint arthritis.[35,36]

Technique
The anterior aspect of the lateral calcaneus is palpated and marked. The incision is created longitudinally superior to the peroneal tendons and below the sinus tarsi.

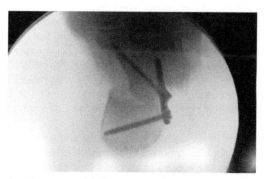

Fig. 15. Alternative fixation can avoid the posterior heel and may allow for more measured medial translation.

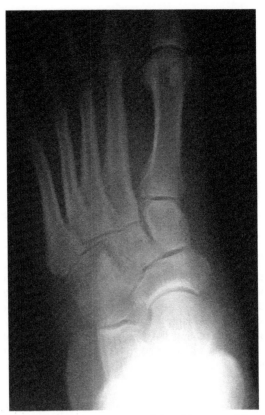

Fig. 16. The Evans calcaneal osteotomy is powerful and is more often used in a transverse plane dominant flatfoot deformity. This foot demonstrates significant talar head uncoverage and calcaneocuboid abduction.

The peroneal tendons are mobilized and retracted plantarly. The osteotomy should be performed 1 to 1.3 cm proximal to the calcaneocuboid joint,[42] and electrocautery can be used to mark the osteotomy. Confirmation of osteotomy location with lateral imaging is recommended.

The osteotomy is made 90° to the long axis of the calcaneus and may angle slightly anteriorly as the osteotomy is deepened. The calcaneocuboid joint should be pinned with a temporary Kirshner wire (K-wire), angled from the cuboid to prevent dorsal translation of the capital fragment of the calcaneus during the opening of the osteotomy. A lamina spreader, pin-based distractor, or specialized spreader is used to pry open the osteotomy and allow correction. Sized spacers are available from multiple companies to allow trialing varying amounts of correction before final fixation. After the placement of the spacer, intraoperative imaging allows the examination of the desired correction by evaluating the talonavicular joint coverage on the dorsoplantar image (**Fig. 17**).

Tricortical allograft and similar grafts can be used and either cut into size or use a precut option. Implants such as porous metal may be chosen as well. The benefit of porous metal implants as there is no absorption that can occur with grafts as they incorporate. The graft should be impacted flush with the lateral wall and not protrude dorsally or plantarly (**Fig. 18**).

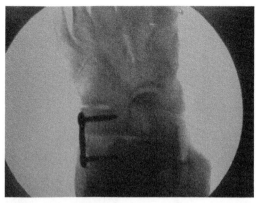

Fig. 17. AP image after the distraction of the calcaneal osteotomy shows good coverage of the talonavicular joint.

The graft or implant typically is stable from the tension the soft issue imparts on the osteotomy. This affords the ability to not fixate the graft or implant. However, if fixation is chosen, plates and screws can be used but may cause peroneal tendon irritation and may need to be removed in the future (**Fig. 19**).

Pearls

- During the osteotomy, the floor of the sinus tarsi can be visualized and care to avoid the middle facet is important.
- Hohmann retractors at the ends of the osteotomy can help protect the soft tissues.
- Caution with an overly stable fixed-angle construct as hardware failure can occur as the graft incorporates and stress is imparted onto the plate.

Calcaneal "Z" Osteotomies

Over the last 20 years, multiple authors have described a "Z" cut calcaneal osteotomy using a single incision that is triplanar. The triplanar nature of this osteotomy allows it

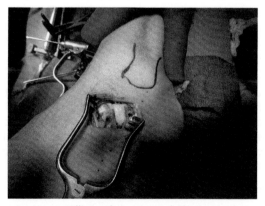

Fig. 18. Whether osseous or metallic wedges are used, the implant or graft must be placed flush.

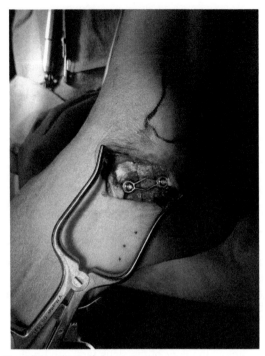

Fig. 19. Plate fixation of the allograft bone wedge.

to achieve similar, but often more, correction than the LCL and MDCO performed independently.[43–46] Today 2 different orientations of the "Z" osteotomies exist, and the first orientation was described by Vander Griend in 2008 as a "Z" osteotomy of the calcaneal neck.[46] The second orientation is described as an extended Z-cut osteotomy[44] (**Fig. 20**).

Indications

Due to the versatility of osteotomies, they can be used for almost any calcaneal correction. True triplane deformity correction is possible, and careful assessment of the needs of the patient is put into osteotomy design. The anterior "Z" allows for increased LCL as wedges can more easily be placed in both vertical arms whereas the extended "Z" wedges are typically only added to the anterior vertical cut.

Technique

Calcaneal exposure for both techniques is relatively the same. An incision is made along the lateral subtalar joint, approximately a centimeter (cm) distal to the posterior inferior aspect of the fibula extending distally to the calcaneal cuboid joint (CCJ). If performing the anterior "Z" osteotomy the incision is cheated anterior to expose the CCJ, whereas with the extended "Z" osteotomy the incision can be cheated slightly posterior. Dissection is carried down, retracting the peroneal tendons, and the lateral calcaneal wall is exposed using a periosteal elevator.

Extended "Z" Osteotomy Cut

Once the lateral calcaneus is exposed the authors like to use K-wires to serve as the 2 apices of the "Z" cut. The first K-wire is typically placed midway between the posterior

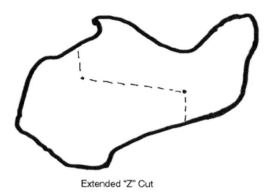

Extended "Z" Cut

Anterior "Z" Cut

Fig. 20. Diagrams illustrating the extended and anterior "Z" cuts.

subtalar joint and the posterior superior tuber of the calcaneus. The wire is then inserted approximately one-third of the way inferior from the superior cortex of the calcaneus. The placement of this wire as it travels lateral to medial is of vital importance.

When planning out the osteotomy cut it is important to think in 3 planes. This osteotomy is unique in that it can correct in all 3 planes. A medial shift is always performed, but how the horizontal arm is cut can determine if the shift is strictly in the transverse plane or if there is a varus tilt to the shift. Cutting from inferior-lateral to superior-medial will produce a varus tilt as the posterior calcaneus is shifted medial. Likewise, it is important not to cut the horizontal arm superior-lateral to inferior-medial as this will maintain a valgus tilt. There can also be the external rotation of the posterior calc to assist in the correction of valgus.

The anterior K-wire is then placed in line with the lateral process of the talus, approximately 2 cm proximal to the calcaneocuboid joint. This wire is placed one-third of the way superior to the plantar cortex of the calcaneus. This anterior wire should be parallel to the posterior wire (**Fig. 21**). Cutting between and parallel to these wires will provide the horizontal arm of the "Z" osteotomy which is typically the first cut performed. Next, directly vertical and perpendicular to the calcaneus cuts are made with the anterior cut extending through the inferior calcaneal cortex and the posterior vertical cut extending through the superior calcaneal cortex (**Fig. 22**).

Anterior "Z" Osteotomy Cut

Once the lateral calcaneus is exposed with proper retraction of the peroneal tendons (which may need to be separated) the cut guides for the anterior "Z" can be placed. K-wires again can be used as the apices, but the authors' preferred method is a pre-made cut guide that hooks into the CCJ laying over the lateral anterior calcaneus. Whichever method is performed to align the cuts, the anterior apex of the "Z" should be 1.3 cm proximal to the CCJ to avoid disrupting the anterior and middle facets when performing the vertical cut.[42] The horizontal cut should be started here and midway between the dorsal and plantar cortex of the anterior calc. The horizontal cut then extends proximally to just anterior to the attachment of the plantar fascia to ensure the vertical cut exiting the plantar cortex does not disrupt ligamentous and muscle attachments. Similar to the extended "Z," the horizontal cut is performed first using the same principles described above to perform either a strictly transverse shift or add varus tilt.

Once the cut is complete an osteotome is used to break through any remaining medial cortex or soft tissue attachments. The use of a lamina spreader or Hintermann distract is used to distract and open the osteotomy while stretching soft tissue attachments. The posterior calcaneus is now shifted medial. The extended "Z" cut does allow for a larger medial shift than the anterior "Z" osteotomy. Once the shift is performed, if LCL is needed then metallic or osseous wedges may be inserted at this time. For the extended "Z," the k-wires for the posterior screws are thrown to stabilize the posterior aspect of the osteotomy and then a Hintermann distractor is used to open the anterior vertical arm for the wedge. Trial sizes are typically used first and on both vertical arms of the anterior "Z" cut and typically only the anterior vertical arm of the extended "Z" (**Fig. 23**). An anterior–posterior radiograph is then taken to ensure proper lengthening of the lateral column is achieved with talonavicular coverage medial.

The extended "Z" osteotomy is routinely fixated with two 4.5 mm to 7.0 mm parallel screws in a similar fashion as any MDCO would be fixated. The wedge placed in the anterior vertical cut is not routinely fixated by the authors as this is inherently stable after posterior compression of the osteotomy is achieved, but a staple or small plate could be applied here for wedge fixation (**Fig. 24**).

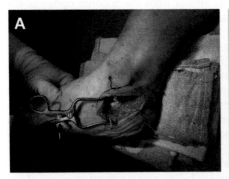 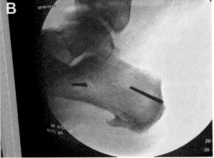

Fig. 21. (*A*, *B*) The anterior K-wire is then placed in line with the lateral process of the talus, approximately 2 cm proximal to the CCJ. This wire is placed one-third of the way superior to the plantar cortex of the calcaneus. This anterior wire should be parallel to the posterior wire. Cutting between and parallel to these wires will provide the horizontal arm of the "Z" osteotomy which is typically the first cut performed.

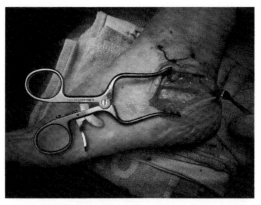

Fig. 22. After completion of all 3 bone cuts, calcaneal translation, rotation, or distraction is possible.

The anterior "Z" osteotomy is fixated with a lateral "Z" plate as the authors preferred method. Due to the anterior nature of the osteotomy, screws are difficult to appropriately position across the entire osteotomy. Another advantage of the plate with the anterior "Z" osteotomy and likely use of wedges in both the anterior and posterior vertical cuts, the lateral "Z" plate allows for fixation across the wedges for added stability (**Fig. 25**).

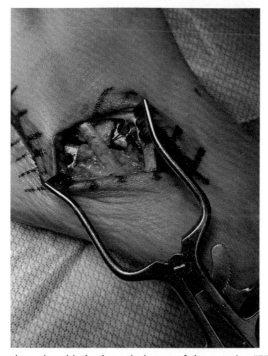

Fig. 23. Metallic wedges placed in both vertical arms of the anterior "Z" cut.

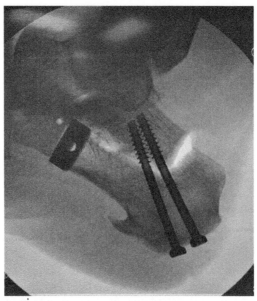

Fig. 24. Fixation of the Extended "Z" cut with press-fit anterior metallic wedge and posterior compression screw placement.

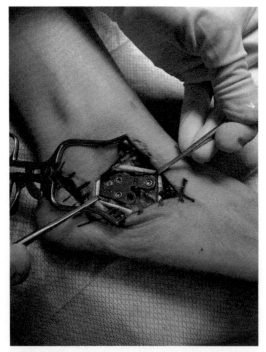

Fig. 25. Lateral "Z" plate fixation of the Anterior "Z" osteotomy can be used due to difficulty with screw placement and for fixation of any wedges that are placed.

Pearls

- Anterior "Z" osteotomy is performed closer to the apex of the lateral column and allows for increased LCL.
- Extended "Z" does allow for wedge placement in the anterior vertical cut to assist in LCL.
- Anterior "Z" provides room for posterior MDCO to assist in posterior calcaneal shift.
- Placement of anterior vertical arm is important in anterior "Z" as to not violate anterior and middle facets.

Cotton Osteotomy

The Cotton opening osteotomy of the medial cuneiform is an important joint sparing adjunctive corrective procedure for forefoot varus. The Cotton osteotomy is a plantarflexory osteotomy of the medial cuneiform which is typically used in the reconstruction of pes planus and PTTD stage II.[47] Cotton in 1936 initially described this opening wedge medial cuneiform osteotomy to restore the "triangle of support."[48] The osteotomy plantar flexes the medial column allowing for the reduction of forefoot varus, recreating the medial longitudinal arch. Providing the correction of forefoot varus deformity through the Cotton osteotomy has been shown to decrease the lateral foot overload that results from persistent forefoot varus and hindfoot alignment is slowly addressed. Advantages of the Cotton osteotomy include the preservation of the metatarsal-cuneiform motion and a predictable union rate.[49]

Scott and colleagues[50] noted that the Cotton osteotomy successfully redistributes the load of the medial column following lengthening of the lateral column in the correction of stage II posterior tibial tendon dysfunction. This makes the Cotton osteotomy a popular adjunctive procedure to the hindfoot osteotomies and tendon rebalancing procedures. Jacobs and Oloff[51] demonstrated excellent results (87.5%) in younger patients (mean age 18.4) following Cotton osteotomy in the combination of medial column procedures for the treatment of congenital painful pes planus. Advantages of the Cotton over first TMT arthrodesis include more predictable union, preservation of first ray mobility, and the ability to vary the amount of correction to restore the "triangle of support" described by Cotton.[52] It is predicted that a surgeon will gain roughly 2.26° of plantar flexion of the medial column for every one-mm graft inserted into the medial cuneiform.[53]

Indications

The Cotton osteotomy is used primarily when the apex of the deformity is located between the first tarsometatarsal joint and naviculocuneiform joint. This osteotomy typically accompanies multiple other surgical procedures including posterior tibialis debridement or advancement, FDL tendon transfer, calcaneal slide osteotomy, and Evans calcaneal osteotomy for the correction of both pediatric and acquired pes planus. A flexible forefoot supination deformity often adequately corrects with a hindfoot reconstructive procedure or either a gastrocnemius recession or tendo-Achilles lengthening. However, if this deformity persists despite these procedures, then a Cotton osteotomy is necessary.[49] This osteotomy is relatively contraindicated in patients with osteoarthritis of the first tarsal-metatarsal (TMT) joint.[54,55] In this case a first TMT arthrodesis may be more beneficial.

Technique

A dorsal incision is created over the medial cuneiform, lateral to the tibialis anterior tendon, and medial to the extensor hallucis longus. The incision is then deepened

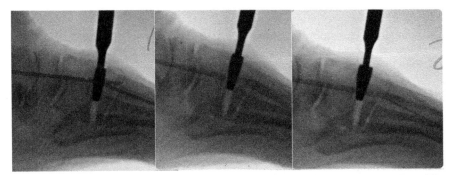

Fig. 26. Correction of the forefoot varus using trial Cotton Osteotomy wedges (4.5–6.5 mm). Each millimeter of the additional wedge should allow for 2.26° of plantar flexion.

down to the medial cuneiform. Identification of the first tarsometatarsal joint as well and the naviculocuneiform joints are completed. The central aspect of the medial cuneiform is marked with the electrocautery. Fluoroscopic examination may be used at this time to ensure appropriate placement. The osteotomy is performed as a midline dorsal to plantar osteotomy through the medial cuneiform, leaving the plantar cortex intact. The osteotomy is then distracted via a lamina spreader or osteotome to stretch the surrounding soft tissue. Trial grafts maybe used to allow for stretching of the soft tissue as well and determining the amount of correction (**Fig. 26**). The appropriately sized bone graft is then inserted maintaining the anticipated correction. Fixation is determined via surgeon preference and comfort level. Other techniques include the use of interpositional plates for the maintenance of the osteotomy[55] (**Fig. 27**).

Pearls

- Expose the first tarsometatarsal joint to ensure appropriate distance from the joint.
- Mobilize the first tarsometatarsal joint to reduce the risk of jamming the joint.
- Use fluoroscopy to identify the correct amount of plantar flexion.
- Use prefabricated Cotton wedges to save time.

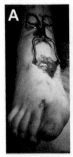
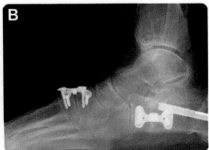
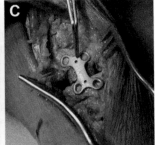

Fig. 27. (*A*) Allograft wedge placed without fixation. (*B*) Dorsal interpositional plate. (*C*) Metallic wedge fixated with a flat plate.

SUMMARY

Flexible PPV deformity is a complicated topic. It requires the surgeon to not only fully recognize and address all levels of deformity and pathology, but then also operate with efficiency to complete all aspects of the reconstruction in one setting. We have presented our most common and powerful techniques, and the indications for them, in the surgical correction of the painful collapsed foot.

DISCLOSURE

J.G. DeVries – Nextremity, Carbofix; DeCarbo – Treace Medical, Smith & Nephew; Scott – Artelon, Avanos, Medline, Parcus, Stryker, Trice; Bussewitz – None; Hyer - Consultant/IP: Integra/Smith-Nephew, CADENCE total ankle replacement.

REFERENCES

1. Johnson KA, Strom DE. Tibialis posterior tendon dysfunction. Clin Orthop Relat Res 1989;239:196–206.
2. Myerson MS. Adult acquired flatfoot deformity: treatment of dysfunction of the posterior tibial tendon. J Bone Joint Surg Am 1996;78-A:780–92.
3. Hill K, Saar WE, Lee TH, et al. Stage II flatfoot: what fails and why. Foot Ankle Clin 2003;8:539–62.
4. Nielsen MD, Dodson EE, Shadrick DL, et al. Nonoperative care for the treatment of adult acquired flatfoot deformity. J Foot Ankle Surg 2011;50:311–4.
5. Kidner FC. The prehallux (accessory scaphoid) in its relation to flat-foot. J Bone Joint Surg 1929;11(4):831–7.
6. Kopp FJ, Marcus RE. Clinical outcome of surgical treatment of the symptomatic accessory navicular. Foot Ankle Int 2004;25(1):27–30.
7. Prichasuk S, Sinphurmsukskul O. Kidner procedure for symptomatic accessory navicular and its relation to pes planus. Foot Ankle Int 1995;16(8):500–3.
8. Choi HJ, Lee WC. Revision surgery for recurrent pain after excision of the accessory navicular and relocation of the tibialis posterior tendon. Clin Orthop Surg 2017;9(2):232–8.
9. Kim J, Day J, Aspang JS. Outcomes following revision surgery after failed Kidner procedure for painful accessory navicular. Foot Ankle Int 2020;41(12):1493–501.
10. Kitaoka HB, Luo ZP, An KN. Effect of the posterior tibial tendon on the arch of the foot during simulated weightbearing: biomechanical analysis. Foot Ankle Int 1997;18(1):43–6.
11. Clarke HD, Kitaoka HB, Ehman RL. Peroneal tendon injuries. Foot Ankle Int 1998; 19(5):280–8.
12. Myerson MS, Badekas A, Schon LC. Treatment of stage II posterior tibial tendon deficiency with flexor digitorum longus tendon and calcaneal osteotomy. Foot Ankle Int 2004;25(7):445–50.
13. Mosier-LaClair S, Pomeroy G, Manoli A. Operative treatment of the difficult stage 2 adult acquired flatfoot deformity. Foot Ankle Clin 2001;6(1):95–119.
14. Den Hartog B. Flexor digitorum longus transfer with medial displacement calcaneal osteotomy. Foot Ankle Clin 2001;6(1):67–76.
15. Aronow MS. Tendon transfer options in managing the adult flexible flatfoot. Foot Ankle Clin 2012;17:205–26.
16. Teasdall RD, Johnson KA. Surgical treatment of stage I posterior tibial tendon dysfunction. Foot Ankle Int 1994;15(12):646–8.

17. Diamond LS, Gould VE. Macrodactyly of the foot: surgical syndactyly after wedge resection. South Med J 1971;67(6):645–50.
18. DiDomenico LA, Thomas ZM, Fahim R. Addressing stage II posterior tibial tendon dysfunction: biomechanically repairing the osseous structures without the need of performing the flexor digitorum longus transfer. Clin Pod Med Surg 2014;31: 391–404.
19. Trevino S, Gould N, Korson R. Surgical treatment of stenosing tenosynovitis at the ankle. Foot Ankle 1981;2(1):37–45.
20. Mosier SM, Lucas DR, Pomeroy G, et al. Pathology of the posterior tibial tendon in posterior tibial tendon insufficiency. Foot Ankle Int 1998;19(8):520–4.
21. Rosenfeld PF, Dick J, Saxby T. The response of the flexor digitorum longus and posterior tibial muscles to tendon transfer and calcaneal osteotomy for stage II posterior tibial tendon dysfunction. Foot Ankle Int 2005;26(9):671–4.
22. Walter JL, Mendicino SS. The flexible adult flatfoot: anatomy and pathome-chanics. Clin Pod Med Surg 2014;31:329–36.
23. Silver RL, de la Garza J, Rang M. The myth of muscle balance: a study of relative strengths and excursions of normal muscles about the foot and ankle. J Bone J Surg 1985;67(3):432–7.
24. Jennings MM, Christiansen JC. The effects of sectioning the spring ligament on rearfoot stability and posterior tibial tendon efficiency. J Foot Ankle Surg 2008; 47(3):219–24.
25. Deland JT, Arnoczky SP, Thompson FM. Adult acquired flatfoot deformity at the talonavicular joint: reconstruction of the spring ligament in an in vitro model. Foot Ankle 1992;13(6):327–32.
26. Nery C, Baumfeld D. Current trends in treatment of injuries to spring ligament. Foot Ankle Clin 2021;26(2):345–59.
27. Deland JT, Ellis SJ, Day J, et al. Indications for deltoid and spring ligament recon-struction in progressive collapsing foot deformity. Foot Ankle Int 2020;41(10): 1302–6.
28. Palmanovish E, Shabat S, Brin YS, et al. Anatomic reconstruction technique for a plantar calcaneonavicular (spring) ligament tear. J Foot Ankle Surg 2015;54(6): 1124–6.
29. Heyes G, Swanton E, Vosoughi AR, et al. Comparative study of spring ligament reconstructions using either hamstring allograft or synthetic ligament augmenta-tion. Foot Ankle Int 2020;41(7):803–10.
30. Tang CYK, Ng KH. A valuable opinion: clinical and radiographic outcomes of braided suture tape system augmentation for spring ligament repair in flexible flatfoot. Foot 2020. https://doi.org/10.1016/j.foot.2020.101685.
31. Koutsogiannis E. Treatment of mobile flat foot by displacement osteotomy of the calcaneus. J Bone Joint Surg Br 1971;53(1):96–100.
32. Myerson MS, Corrigan J, Thompson F, et al. Tendon transfer combined with calcaneal osteotomy for treatment of posterior tibialis tendon insufficiency: a radiographic investigation. Foot Ankle Int 1995;16(11):712–8.
33. Myerson MS, Fortin P, Cunningham B. Changes in tibiotalar contact with calca-neal osteotomy. Trans Am Acad Orthop Surg 1994;61:149.
34. Guyton GP, Jeng C, Krieger LE, et al. Flexor digitorum longus transfer and medial displacement calcaneal osteotomy for posterior tibial tendon dysfunction: a middle-term clinical follow-up. Foot Ankle Int 2001;22:627–32.
35. Marks RM, Long JT, Ness ME, et al. Surgical reconstruction of posterior tibial tendon dysfunction: prospective comparison of flexor digitorum longus

substitution combined with lateral column lengthening or medial displacement calcaneal osteotomy. Gait Posture 2009;29:17–22.

36. Bolt PM, Coy S, Toolan BC. A comparison of lateral column lengthening and medial translation osteotomy of the calcaneus for the reconstruction of adult acquired flatfoot. Foot Ankle Int 2007;28:1115–23.

37. Evans D. Calcaneo-valgus deformity. J Bone Joint Surg Br 1975;57(3):270–8.

38. Dolan CM, Henning JA, Anderson JG, et al. Randomized prospective study comparing tri-cortical iliac crest autograft to allograft in the lateral column lengthening component for operative correction of adult acquired flatfoot deformity. Foot Ankle Int 2007;28:8–12.

39. Grier KM, Walling AK. The use of tricortical autograft versus allograft in lateral column lengthening for adult acquired flatfoot deformity: an analysis of union rate and complications. Foot Ankle Int 2010;31:760–9.

40. Cooper PS, Nowak M, Shaer J. Calcaneocuboid joint pressures with lateral column lengthening (Evans) procedure. Foot Ankle Int 1997;18:199–205.

41. Momberger N, Morgan JM, Bachus KN, et al. Calcaneocuboid joint pressure after lateral column lengthening in a cadaveric planovalgus deformity model. Foot Ankle Int 2000;21:730–5.

42. Hyer CF, Lee T, Block AJ, et al. Evaluation of the anterior and middle talocalcaneal articular facets and the Evans osteotomy. J Foot Ankle Surg 2002;41(6):389–93.

43. Demetracopulos CA, Nair P, Malzberg A, et al. Outcomes of a stepcut lengthening calcaneal osteotomy for adult acquired flatfoot deformity. Foot Ankle Int 2015;36(7):749–55.

44. Ebaugh MP, Larson DR, Reb CW, et al. Outcomes of the extended Z-cut osteotomy for correction of adult acquired flatfoot defomrity. Foot Ankle Int 2019;40(8):914–22.

45. Scott RT, Berlet GC. Calcaneal Z osteotomy for extra-articular correction of hindfoot valgus. J Foot Ankle Surg 2013;52(3):406–8.

46. Vander Griend R. Lateral column lengthening using a "Z" osteotomy of the calcaneus. Tech Foot Ankle Surg 2008;7(4):257–63.

47. Yarmel D, Mote G, Treaster A. The Cotton osteotomy: a technical guide. J Foot Ankle Surg 2009;48(4):506–12.

48. Cotton FJ. Foot statics and surgery. N Eng J Med 1936;214:24–7.

49. Tankson CJ. The Cotton osteotomy: indications and techniques. Foot Ankle Clin 2007;12:309–15.

50. Scott AT, Hendry TM, Iaquinto JM, et al. Plantar pressure analysis in cadaver feet after bony procedures commonly used in the treatment of stage II posterior tibial tendon insufficiency. Foot Ankle Int 2007;28:1143–53.

51. Jacobs AM, Oloff LM. Surgical management of forefoot supinatus in flexible flatfoot deformity. J Foot Ankle Surg 1984;23:410–9.

52. Hirose CB, Johnson JE. Plantarflexion opening wedge medial cuneiform osteotomy for correction of fixed forefoot varus associated with flatfoot deformity. Foot Ankle Int 2004;25(8):568–74.

53. Scott RT, Bussewitz BW, Hyer CF, et al. The corrective power of the cotton osteotomy. FussSprungg 2016;14:9–13.

54. Coughlin MJ, Mann RA, Saltzman CL. Surgery of the foot and ankle. 8th edition. Philadelphia, PA: Mosby Inc; 2007. p. 1047–58.

55. League AC, parks BG, Schon LC. Radiographic and pedobarographic comparison of femoral head allograft versus block plate with dorsal opening wedge medial cuneiform osteotomy: a biomechanical study. Foot Ankle Int 2008;29(9):922–6.

Deformity Correction of the Midfoot/Hindfoot/Ankle

Ryan T. Scott, DPM[a],*, Michael D. Dujela, DPM[b], Jason George DeVries, DPM[c], Christopher F. Hyer, DPM, MS[d,e], Travis Langan, DPM[f], Mark A. Prissel, DPM[d,e], Bryan Van Dyke, DO[g]

KEYWORDS

- Hindfoot fusion • Ankle fusion • Tibiotalocalcaneal fusion • Posttraumatic arthritis
- Medial double

KEY POINTS

- The authors discuss the reconstructive options for repair of the deformed/arthritic midfoot, hindfoot, and ankle
- Joint destruction surgery requires a comprehensive approach to the entire deformity, we care to address the mechanical, bony, and soft tissue concerns
- The authors discuss the rational for procedure choice, as well as techniques and pearls for the surgical procedures

'Midfoot FLATFOOT- NC, 2nd/3rd TMT FUSION
Indications

Pes planovalgus deformity is typically a combined hindfoot and forefoot deformity.[1] When evaluating a flatfoot deformity it is important to appropriately identify the axis of deformity. The plane of deformity will greatly influence the surgical procedures warranted to manage the instability. In the flatfoot deformity, the forefoot abducts and the medial arch collapses. Oftentimes, the deformity maybe distal to the talonavicular (TN) joint (IE: naviculocuneiform joint (NCJ)/tarsometatarsal joints (TMTJs)).[1] Evaluation of

[a] Board Certified, Foot & Ankle Reconstructive Surgery, The CORE Institute Foot and Ankle Reconstruction Fellowship, The CORE Institute, 9321 West Thomas Road, Suite 205, Phoenix, AZ 85037, USA; [b] Board Certified, Foot & Ankle Reconstructive Surgery, Advanced Foot and Ankle Surgical Fellowship, Washington Orthopaedic Center, 1900 Crooks Hill Road, Centralia, WA 98531, USA; [c] Board Certified, Foot & Ankle Reconstructive Surgery, Orthopedics & Sports Medicine – BayCare Clinic, 501 North 10th Street, Manitowoc, WI 54220, USA; [d] Board Certified, Foot & Ankle Reconstructive Surgery, Orthopedic Foot & Ankle Center, Columbus, OH, USA; [e] Orthopedic Foot & Ankle Center, 350 West Wilson Bridge Road, Suite 200, Worthington, OH 43085, USA; [f] Board Certified, Foot and Ankle Reconstructive Surgery, Carle Orthopedics and Sports Medicine, Champaign, IL 61820, USA; [g] Summit Orthopaedics, 2321 Coronado Street, Idaho Falls, ID 83404, USA
* Corresponding author.
E-mail address: scottryt@gmail.com

Clin Podiatr Med Surg 39 (2022) 233–272
https://doi.org/10.1016/j.cpm.2021.11.011
0891-8422/22/© 2021 Elsevier Inc. All rights reserved.

the midfoot may demonstrate a fault secondary to laxity or sometimes rigid deformity is noted. Arthrodesis of the naviculocuneiform and TMTJs allows for increased stability as well as deformity correction in the flatfoot deformity especially when soft tissue rebalancing is not an option.[2–6] (**Figs. 1** and **2**)

Management of the flatfoot deformity is performed in a very strategic stepwise approach. The hindfoot is addressed initially working from proximal to distal. After the realignment of the hindfoot, attention is directed to the midfoot. Incisional placement for midfoot fusions varies depending on the joints involved. If the NCJ is the only joint that requires attention, the incision can be placed either medial or dorsal. Adequate joint exposure can be achieved with either approach. The medial incision may not allow for full access to the lateral cuneiform joint; however, the medial and central cuneiform joint surfaces allow for adequate fusion and stability of the joint.[3] When an isolated NC joint fusion is required, we recommend the dorsal approach.

When addressing the instability of the TMTJs, several approaches have been described. Typically, a dorsomedial incision over the first TMTJs is preferred. This allows for appropriate visualization of the joint as well as leaving and appropriate skin bridge for other midfoot fusions. When a second and third TMT joint fusion is planned, the incision is positioned over the lateral aspect of the second metatarsal base.

INSTRUMENTS

Pin distractor, lamina spreader, curette, osteotomes, rotary bur, solid drill bit.

TECHNIQUE

Depending on the desired approach, a medial or dorsal incision is created. The medial incision is placed between the tibialis anterior (TA) and tibialis posterior tendon. Care is taken to protect these tendons throughout the surgical procedure. Dissection can then be taken quickly down to the NCJ. The medial saphenous nerve may be encountered at the distal aspect of the incision. This is retracted plantar and a capsular incision is made exposing the medial aspect of the NC joint.

With the dorsal approach, a dorsal incision is placed in the interval between the TA and extensor hallucis longus (EHL) tendon. Again, care is taken to protect the tendinous structures throughout the case. Dissection is carried through the soft tissue.

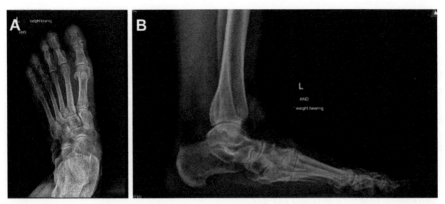

Fig. 1. (A–B): Weight-bearing AP and lateral radiograph demonstrating forefoot abduction and instability of the medial column.

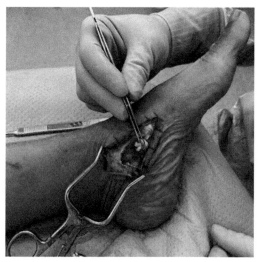

Fig. 2. A full-thickness tear of the posterior tibial tendon.

The neurovascular bundle will be just lateral to the EHL. As long as this is visualized and the dissection remains medial, full-thickness dissection can be performed. A capsular incision will show the central aspect of the NC joint. A small Cobb elevator or wide Key elevator is used to free the remaining capsule allowing for full visualization.

If the second and third TMTJs are involved, a dorsal incision can be carried distal to expose the TMT joints. The deep neurovascular bundle is protected medially. The use of fluoroscopy can aid in incisional placement.

Once the respective joint is identified, a pin distractor is used to allow access for adequate joint preparation. With the joint distracted an osteotomy is gently passed into and around the joint to ensure appropriate release and mobilization of the joint. The cartilage is then meticulously denuded using surgeon preference. We prefer a curette, osteotomes, and a rongeur. A resurfacing tool (bur) can also be used to ensure full removal of the cartilage and debridement of the subchondral plate. The joint surfaces are then fenestrated with a solid drill bit and an osteotome. Bone graft or biologics can be placed into the joint if necessary or desired. After joint preparation, manual reduction is used to correct the deformity. A large retractor (Army Navy) applying plantar to dorsal force on the navicular can assist sagittal plane correction. Temporary fixation is placed stabilizing the joint and maintaining the reduction. Fluoroscopic examination is then performed to verify adequate deformity correction. Multiple fixation methods are available for NC and TMT fusions. Fixation options range from screws, plates, staples, or a combination of the above. Grossman and colleagues described an all-screw fixation construct for NC joint fusions demonstrating appropriate stability and fusion rates. Strategic screw placement allows for cross-screws stacked above each other. Locking and nonlocking plate options are available as well. Care must be taken not to violate the TA tendon insertion with plate fixation. **Figs. 3–6**.

Many midfoot fusions may need to be carried to the TMTJs as well. If the deformity continues to the TMTJ or the TMTJ is also arthritic, the joint complex should also be included. Joint prep and deformity correction are similar as described for the NC joint. Fixation constructs also vary, but with limited real estate, screw/staple combinations can be quick and effective. **Figs. 7** and **8**.

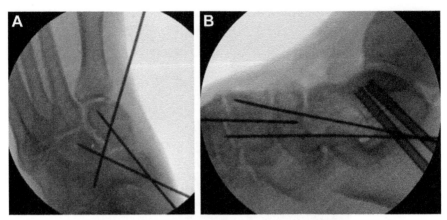

Fig. 3. (A, B): Reduction and placement of the temporary guidewires across the NC joint within multiple planes.

POSTOP PROTOCOL

NC and TMT fusion(s) in the management of flatfoot deformity are often combined with other soft tissue and osseous procedures. The larger fusions will take priority over the midfoot fusions and often dictate the postoperative course. If the midfoot fusions are the driving force, we recommend 1 to 2 weeks in a postoperative splint. Ice and elevation will significantly help in the reduction of postoperative swelling. Sutures/staples will be removed at the first postop appointment pending skin healing. Transition into a non–weight-bearing cast is performed for the next 4 weeks. Radiographs attained at the 6-week mark will determine transition into a cam walking boot or short leg walking cast. Ideally, a cam walking boot is applied, and physical therapy is initiated. Ten-week postop radiographs are once again obtained. Pending the consolidation of the fusions, transition into regular shoe gear is performed.

COMPLICATIONS

Some of the potential complications of the NC/TMT fusion include: neurovascular injury, jamming of the adjacent joints due to under/over correction, hardware pain, mal-union, nonunion.

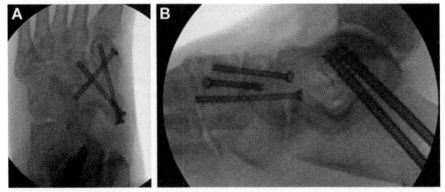

Fig. 4. (A, B): Intraoperative lateral and AP radiographs demonstrating stacked screw construct for NC arthrodesis.

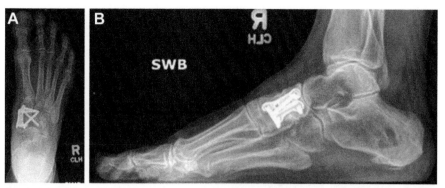

Fig. 5. (*A, B*): Medially placed locking plate with cross-screw fixation for NC joint arthrodesis.

PEARLS

- Preoperative planning is important for incision placement
- Identification and retraction of the neurovascular bundle
- Use of a pin distractor to get adequate visualization
- Rigid stable fixation of the joints
- Fuse the joints from proximal to distal

MEDIAL APPROACH DOUBLE (TALONAVICULAR SUBTALAR JOINT)
Background

Correction of adult-acquired flatfoot, rigid deformity, or arthritic hindfoot joints can be accomplished with hindfoot fusion surgeries. The triple arthrodesis has long been a

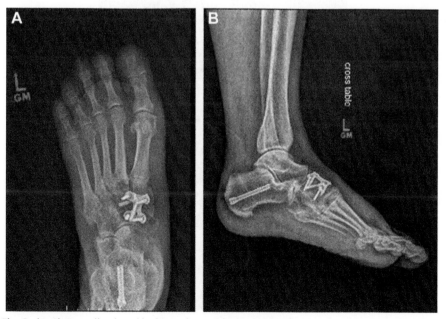

Fig. 6. (*A, B*): Dorsally placed locking plate with cross-screw fixation for NC joint arthrodesis. Medial displacement calcaneal slide osteotomy performed.

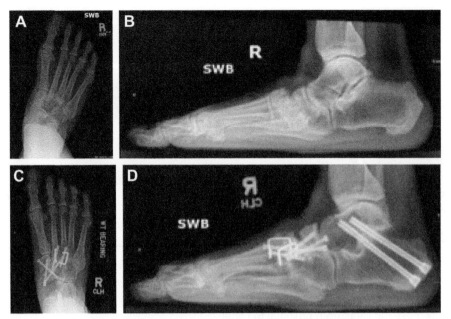

Fig. 7. (*A, B*) Preoperative lateral and AP foot demonstrating NC joint fault with underlying flatfoot deformity. (*C, D*) Postoperative lateral and AP demonstrating flatfoot correction with multiple joint arthrodesis (STJ, NC, and TMT joints).

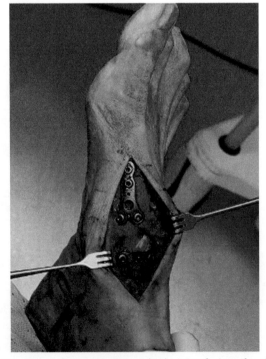

Fig. 8. Intraoperative image demonstrating multiple joint fusions for the correction of a flatfoot deformity (TN and 1st TMT joints).

procedure for the management of these issues, but more recently the double arthrodesis has been advocated, sparing the calcanealcuboid joint.[6–13] The double arthrodesis has been shown to be safe and effective for hindfoot deformity correction.[6–14] This can be performed through a 2 incision technique with one lateral and one dorsal, or through one incision on the medial side of the foot. Correction of a large valgus deformity may leave the lateral skin under tension and wound healing complications have been reported.[13] With the proper technique, the procedure can be performed safely and effectively through a single medial incision.[6–13] Indications for a single medial incision approach to a double arthrodesis include any patient with high-risk wound complications who may need a realignment arthrodesis.[6–13] Surgeons may also choose this technique for its ease of exposure and closure.

Instruments

Pin distractor, lamina spreader, curette, osteotomes, rotary bur, solid drill bit.

Technique

This technique accomplished through a single medial incisional approach. The incision is placed from the tip of the medial malleolus to just distal to the navicular tuberosity. The interval between the TA and tibial posterior tendons is used. After skin incision, the subcutaneous tissue is divided. Care is taken to avoid the saphenous vein and individual branches are cauterized to maintain hemostasis. The saphenous nerve is also avoided in the subcutaneous tissue along the superior margin of the incision. The navicular tuberosity is identified with the insertion of the posterior tibial tendon. The TN joint capsule is identified and incised to allow joint exposure (**Figs. 9–12**).

The dissection is carried posteriorly to expose the subtalar joint (STJ). The spring ligament is divided if present. Often the spring ligament is torn and retracted from chronic pes planovalgus foot alignment. The sustentaculum tali is identified on the

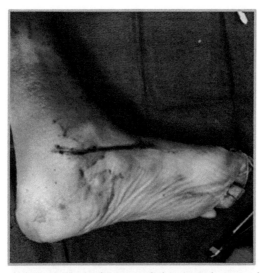

Fig. 9. A recommended "Lazy S" curvilinear medial incisional approach from the inferior aspect of the medial malleolus down over the sustentaculum tali and dorsal over the medial aspect of the talonavicular joint.

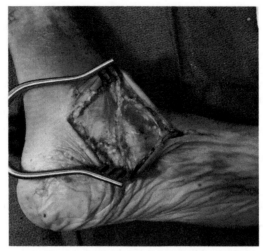

Fig. 10. Subcutaneous exposure to the level of the posterior tibial tendon sheath.

calcaneus and the STJ is identified superior to this landmark. The medial neurovascular bundle is avoided and protected as it passes inferior to the sustentaculum tali, beneath the posterior tibial tendon. The posterior tibial tendon may be chronically torn and degenerative. Diseased distal posterior tendon can be transected and allowed to retract into the retromalleolar space if deemed to be nonviable for repair. Additionally, a flexor digitorum longus tendon transfer may be incorporated into the navicular after joint fixation to aid in foot adduction and medial ankle support. The deltoid ligament complex is carefully peeled away from the medial wall of the talus and calcaneus. It is important to repair this tissue on closure to avoid postoperative valgus ankle collapse. The STJ capsule is incised and the joint exposed. The middle and

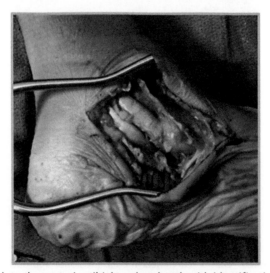

Fig. 11. Exposure into the posterior tibial tendon sheath with identification of the posterior tibial tendon (superior) and the FDL tendon (inferior).

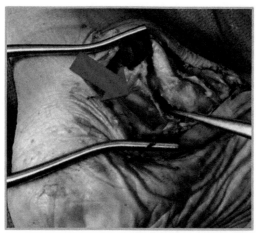

Fig. 12. Self-retaining retraction creating a "safe zone" with the posterior tibial tendon retracted superiorly and the FDL retracted inferiorly. Note the arrow indicating the sustentaculum tali to aid in identifying the level of the middle facet of the subtalar joint.

posterior facets are visualized. It is useful to make sure that the joints are adequately released and able to be reduced into appropriate alignment for fusion. Joint contractures and exostosis may need to be released to allow appropriate joint position for fusion. A percutaneous posterior muscle group release is often performed to allow appropriate correction of the STJ.

A lamina spreader or a Hintermann retractor is useful to individually distract the TN and STJs. The remaining cartilage of both joints is thoroughly removed using surgeon's preference of instruments, typically osteotomes and curettes. The joints are irrigated and suctioned to remove loose debris. The joint surfaces of the navicular, talus, and calcaneus are fenestrated with a drill bit and roughened further with osteotome fish-scaling technique. Meticulous removal of cartilage and sclerotic subchondral bone to expose healthy subchondral bone is paramount for achieving solid bone fusion. Bone autograft or bone marrow aspirate may be added to the fusion sites to further signal for bone healing. The author's preferred source is calcaneal bone autograft harvested from a separate small lateral calcaneal tuberosity incision using a bone graft harvesting reamer. Biologic adjuvants such as platelet-derived growth factor may be added to the fusion sites at this time as well.

With the joints well prepared and the autograft/biologics place, the joints are reduced into the neutral position and pinned with guidewire for cannulated screws. The STJ is reduced first and care is taken to achieve neutral or very slight valgus at the STJ. Inadequate correction of hindfoot valgus will lead to ongoing pain and valgus stress on the ankle. One or 2 guidewires for 6.5 to 7.5 mm cannulated screws are placed from the posterior tuberosity of the calcaneus to the talar body. Wire placement is confirmed with fluoroscopy, especially lateral and Harris axial views. An AP ankle view is useful to make sure the end of the screw will be central in the talus. The ideal wire starting point should avoid the plantar weight-bearing aspect of the calcaneus to reduce uncomfortable screw head position necessitating subsequent hardware removal. It is useful to provisionally pin the TN joint at this time to ensure appropriate foot alignment can be achieved. The talar head should be fully covered on the AP fluoroscopic view and Meary's angle should be neutral from the talus into the first metatarsal (**Figs. 13–16**).

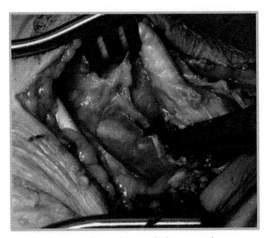

Fig. 13. Exposing the subtalar joint from the medial approach.

The skin is incised off the subtalar wire and a hemostat is used to dissect down to bone. A variety of cannulated screws are available. Headless screws are able to be buried further into the bone and avoid prominent calcaneal hardware. A countersink is used and the screw length is measured. A drill is used to at least open the near cortex. Based on the patient's bone density, the drill may need to be passed across the joint even with self-drilling, self-tapping screws. Strong joint compression should be felt like the screw head seats in the bone. Fluoroscopy is used to make sure the dorsal surface of the talus is not violated and there is no prominent hardware.

With the STJ compressed and fixated, the foot is evaluated to make sure the TN joint is still in a good position. Pronation and supination through the Chopart joints may need to be adjusted to create a plantigrade foot. Fixation across the TN joint can be achieved with screws, staples, or plate fixation. Typically, 2 or 3 cannulated 5.5 mm

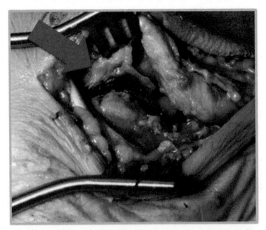

Fig. 14. Soft tissue (deltoid ligament – indicated by the *arrow*) reflected from sustentaculum tali to aid in improved visualization and exposure of the posterior facet of the subtalar joint (Note: the deltoid ligament requires repair back to the sustentaculum tali at the completion of the procedure).

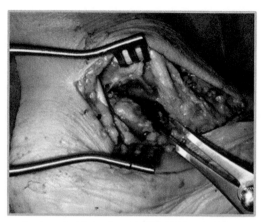

Fig. 15. Laminar spreader inserted into the subtalar joint providing excellent visualization to the posterior facet of the subtalar joint for joint preparation.

screws are used percutaneously across the TN joint and can be supplemented with staple or plate fixation as needed. The first wire goes from the navicular tuberosity into the talar neck parallel with the axis of the talus. The second and third wires go from dorsal navicular into the talar neck. Care is taken to avoid the dorsal pedal artery during the placement of this wire. Wire position may need to be adjusted to avoid the subtalar fusion hardware. Screw placement is similar to the subtalar fusion with head-less screws often used to avoid prominent screw heads. However, headed screws or even washers may be useful for poor navicular bone quality (see **Figs. 1** and **2**).

The subalar and TN joints should now be compressed and fixated with an appropriate alignment of the patient's foot. The deltoid ligament complex is repaired with 0-vicryl suture. This is critical to avoiding postoperative valgus ankle collapse. An FDL tendon transfer to the navicular is performed if desired. The subcutaneous layer is closed with 2 to 0 vicryl suture and the skin is closed with nylon suture. The tourniquet is deflated during closure to ensure there is adequate hemostasis. A well-padded

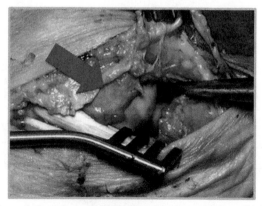

Fig. 16. Visualization of the talonavicular joint with the posterior tibial tendon retracted inferiorly providing excellent visualization of the talonavicular joint for preparation (Note – arrow indicating tibiospring portion of the deltoid ligament which requires repair to the navicular at the completion of the case.

posterior splint is placed with the ankle at the neutral position to prevent equinus contracture (**Fig. 17**).

Postop Protocol

Patient is kept non–weight-bearing on the operative foot. The splint is removed at 1 week and short leg cast is placed. The sutures are removed when skin heals usually 2 to 3 weeks after surgery. The patient is kept non–weight-bearing in a removable boot until about 8 weeks after surgery based on follow-up radiographs. Patient is then weight-bearing as tolerated in the boot until about 12 weeks after surgery. Physical therapy is used as need to work on ankle range of motion, strengthening, and gait training.

TALONAVICULAR MEDIAL, SUBTALAR JOINT LATERAL, TRADITIONAL FUSIONS
Indications

Traditional arthrodesis of one or several joints of the hindfoot can be undertaken in similar indications to medial approach arthrodesis. All conservative measures should have been undertaken, and the pathology should not be correctable with a less restrictive operation. If the pathology can be corrected adequately with osteotomy work or

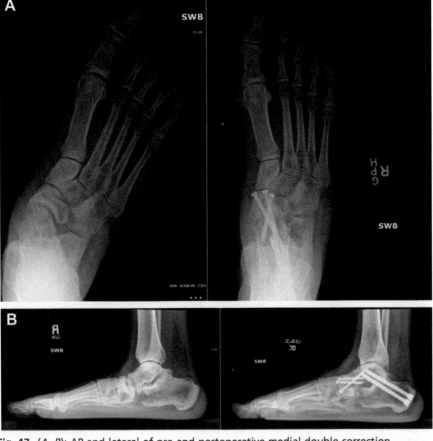

Fig. 17. (A, B): AP and lateral of pre and postoperative medial double correction.

isolated arthrodesis, this should be given priority. If realignment arthrodesis is indicated, both medial approach and traditional incision arthrodesis have been shown to correct malalignment.[7]

A few specific indications can be outlined. In the case of isolated arthritis with minimal deformity of either the TN or STJs, isolated fusion of these joints will have the advantage to preserve other motion segments. An isolated STJ fusion is further indicated in talocalcaneal coalition with adaptive changes, sinus tarsi syndrome, and posttraumatic arthritis, particularly regarding joint depression type calcaneal fractures.[15–17] An isolated TN joint fusion can be after the specific fracture of the talus or navicular leading to posttraumatic arthritis or collapse through the joint. Mueller–Weiss syndrome is a condition for which the navicular bone goes through spontaneous avascular necrosis, and this may necessitate fusion of the TN joint with or without incorporation of the NCJ.[18–20] The traditional 2-incision triple arthrodesis may also be indicated over a medial double arthrodesis in several instances. This includes in cases of true and significant calcaneocuboid arthritis and in cases such as a cavus foot in which shortening of the lateral column is beneficial. The triple may also be used in cases whereby added construct stability may be desired such as revision surgery, obesity, or poor bone quality.

Dorsal talonavicular joint arthrodesis technique

The dorsal incision is straight and located along the TA tendon. Typically, this will run along the medial border of the tibialis tendon in a valgus deformity due to the external rotation of the forefoot, and lateral in a cavus deformity. Dissection is carried deeply adjacent to the TA tendon, either medial or lateral depending on foot structure. A linear capsulotomy is then used from the ankle joint and onto the navicular body. Exposure of the TN joint is then carried out medially and laterally.

Joint preparation must be meticulous and carried out on both sides of the joint. The talar head is exposed with the use of a small joint distractor or can be exposed and elevated by placing a Cobb elevator into the joint and dislocating the talar head out of the joint. The articular surface is completely denuded of the articular surface and should be carried deep to the subchondral plate. Once this is performed, the joint surface is fenestrated with a large bore guidewire or small drill, and the joint surface is fish scaled with a $^1/_4$" osteotome. The undersurface of the navicular joint is more difficult due to the shape of the joint. Typically, a small osteotome and angled curette are needed. Again, after cartilage removal, fenestration and fish scaling are performed.

Once prepared, the area may be packed with autogenous graft or orthobiologic options. The joint is aligned as needed and held into place. Once aligned, a guidewire for a 4.0 to 5.0 mm cannulated screw is driven percutaneously into the plantar distal portion of the navicular tuberosity and placed in a lateral and dorsal direction into the talus. Position should be held, and a second wire is placed dorsally from the center-lateral aspect of the navicular into the talus either parallel to the plantar aspect of the foot or slightly plantar. Care is taken not to project into the STJ as this will restrict the positioning of the STJ. In almost all cases 45 mm screws will be used to cross the TN joint and obtain good purchase in the talus without extending into other joints. The plantar-medial screw is countersunk, but the dorsal screw does not require this. These are placed in lag technique and usually partially threaded screws are used. This is confirmed with intraoperative fluoroscopy.

Lateral subtalar joint arthrodesis technique

A longitudinal incision is made from the distal tip of the fibula to the base of the fourth metatarsal. Dissection is carried deep with care taken to avoid injury to the sural nerve in the inferior flap. The extensor digitorum brevis (EDB) muscle belly is identified, and the peroneal tendons are protected. A large Weitlaner or Gelpi retractor is placed to maintain retraction of the wound edges. The deep fascia over the EDB muscle is incised, and the muscle belly is sharply elevated off the calcaneus using a #15 scalpel to expose the sinus tarsi. The soft tissues of the sinus tarsi obscure visibility of the middle and posterior facets of the STJ and are removed with a rongeur. A lamina spreader can be placed at this point into the joint between the talar head and anterior process of the calcaneus. Once in place, the lamina spreader can be opened maximally. This will expose the posterior facet of the STJ. Initially, a curved 1/2″ osteotome is used to remove the articular surfaces of the calcaneus and talus. A rongeur is used to remove debris and any impinging osteophytes. The posterior curvature of the calcaneal articular surface is cleared with an angled curette. Again, after cartilage removal, fenestration and fish scaling are performed.(**Figs. 18–37**)

Once prepared, the area is packed with autogenous bone graft or orthobiologics. A combination of rotation and sliding of the talus relative to the calcaneus is performed to realign the STJ. The optimum position is neutral to slightly valgus alignment of the hindfoot. A guidewire for a 6.5 to 7.0 mm is inserted into the posterior inferior aspect of the calcaneus and advanced just through the posterior facet articular surface whereby placement can be confirmed under direct visualization. Once the satisfactory trajectory is confirmed, the wire is advanced to the subchondral bone at the talar dome. The posterior heel has a stab incision over the guidewire and the area is drilled. Counter sinking of a headed screw should be undertaken to avoid prominence at the weight-bearing surface of the heel. The appropriately sized screw should be selected with care taken to ensure there is sufficient clearance of all screw threads across the joint to avoid distraction force which may result in gapping at the joint surface. A second screw is generally placed to add additional compression and to provide an antirotation effect.

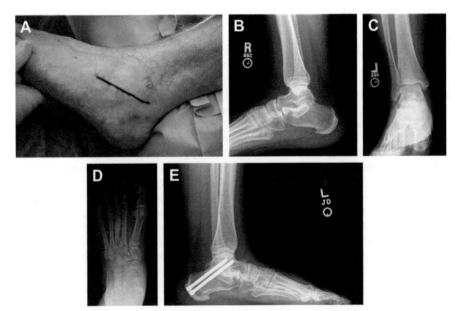

Fig. 18. (A–E): The proposed incision from the distal fibula to the level of the fourth metatarsal base crossing the sinus tarsi.

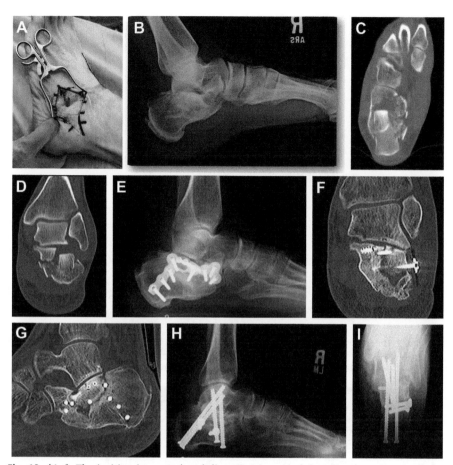

Fig. 19. (*A–I*): The incision is created and dissection is carried down to the extensor digitorum brevis muscle. A self-retaining retractor is used.

Traditional triple arthrodesis technique

In cases of a traditional 2-incision triple arthrodesis, the lateral incision will be lengthened to expose the calcaneocuboid joint. The CC joint is prepared in a similar fashion. Instead of a lamina spreader in the joint, a small joint wire distractor, such as a Hintermann retractor, is used to open and expose the joint. The joint has a saddle shape and the deep aspects of the joint are sometimes difficult to fully expose. In addition, the use of a 1/4″ osteotome may be preferred due to the small size and curvature of the joint. Conversely, a sagittal saw can be used to resect the joint surfaces. This will result in more shortening than debridement and curettage of the joint and should be reserved for cavus foot types that can benefit from this shortening. Joint fenestration and fish scaling are undertaken again.

Fixation in a traditional triple arthrodesis is similar. Typically, the TN joint is pinned first, then the STJ. With the combined arthrodesis, a screw in the STJ from the top down may be considered due to the ease of access and orientation. Once pinned into place, the TN joints are fixated first. Finally, a lateral plate (such as a 4-hole H-plate style) is used to fixate the CC joint. Most plates can be placed with eccentric drilling of the screws to allow for compression of the joint through the plate. Very little motion is

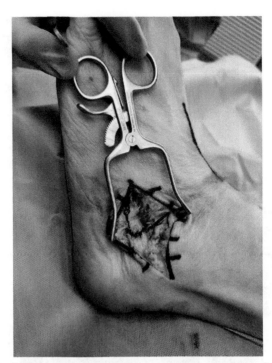

Fig. 20. Incision is planned to elevate the EDB muscle from the floor of the sinus tarsi.

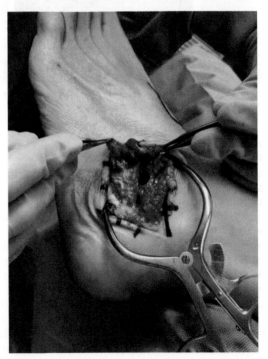

Fig. 21. Elevation of EDB muscle belly from the sinus tarsi to enhance visualization and access to the subtalar joint.

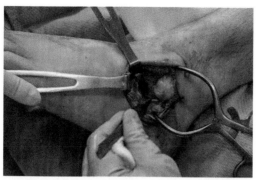

Fig. 22. After the contents of the sinus tarsi are removed, the anterior aspect of the posterior facet is now readily visualized.

present at the CC joint after the TN and STJs are fixated, and all that is usually needed is pressure plantar to the cuboid bone to avoid subluxation.

ANTERIOR APPROACH ANKLE FUSION
Indications

Ankle arthrodesis has long been the gold standard for the management of deformity and osteoarthritis of the tibiotalar joint. Ankle arthrodesis has been described to have high patient outcome scores with low complication rates. Ankle arthrodesis historically has roughly a 13% incidence of nonunion.[21] Traditionally performed with screws, the anterior ankle arthrodesis has gained significant headway due to advancing plating systems and technology. With the transition to anatomically contoured single column anterior ankle arthrodesis plates improved outcomes have been demonstrated in the literature reducing the nonunion rate to 4.5%, according to soon to be published systematic review involving 357 ankles from 15 publications (data on file).[22] Although, ankle arthroplasty is beginning to become more popular and successful in patients with ankle arthritis, is substantial cohort still exist that is not an appropriate candidate for arthroplasty, for reasons including compromised bone stock, prior infection, severe malalignment, avascular necrosis, compromised soft tissue envelope, and peripheral neuropathy among other etiologies.

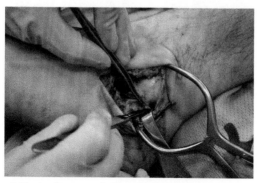

Fig. 23. The calcaneal fibular ligament is identified and released to facilitate visualization and prep of the posterior facet.

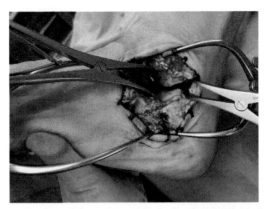

Fig. 24. Excellent visualization of the calcaneal and talar components of the posterior facet with joint release and dual lamina spreaders.

Some of the greatest advantages of the anterior ankle joint arthrodesis include visualization of both malleoli, ease of joint preparation, as well as deformity management. As the popularity of total ankle replacement (TAR) increases, the anterior approach ankle fusion has also gained popularity. Surgeons are becoming more familiar and comfortable with the dissection and the structures at risk during this procedure. Although alternate approaches exist including lateral with fibular takedown, posterior,

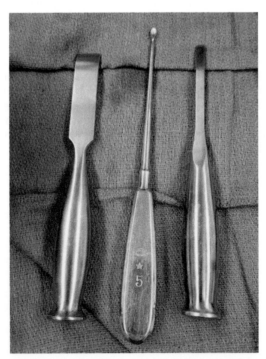

Fig. 25. Instrument sequence for cartilage removal- ½ inch curved Smith Peterson osteotome followed by small curette and ¼ inch curved osteotome for "fish scaling".

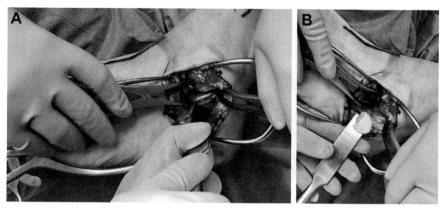

Fig. 26. (*A, B*): A ½ inch curved osteotome facilitates rapid removal of large segments of cartilage.

and arthroscopic our preference is for the malleolar sparing direct anterior approach and we encourage surgeons to spare the malleoli whenever possible.

Instruments

Pin distractor, lamina spreader, curettes, osteotomes, rotary bur, solid drill bit, sagittal saw, bone graft, arthrodesis hardware.

Technique

An anterior incision is placed central across the ankle in between the TA and EHL. A rough estimate of the incision length is 3 finger breathes below the tibiotalar joint and 4 finger breathes above. This will provide the novice surgeon with a good starting point. The incision is then deepened down to the extensor retinaculum. Sharp incision through the retinaculum is then performed. "Tag sutures" are then placed in the retinaculum to assist in retraction as well as to assist in closure at the end of the case. Sharp dissection is then performed lateral to the TA tendon, ensuring the TA to remain within its sheath. The neurovascular bundle will be retracted laterally out of the way with large retraction. We prefer Army Navy retractors during this time. Several transverse vessels will be noted superior to the ankle joint capsule. Electrocautery is

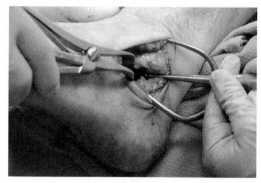

Fig. 27. A curette is used to remove remaining cartilage followed by copious saline irrigation to remove remnants that could impair healing.

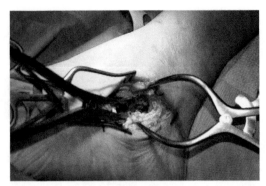

Fig. 28. An extensive grid pattern is created via subchondral drilling to both the calcaneal and talar subtalar joint surfaces.

used to hemostasis control of these vessels. A full-thickness incision is then made through the ankle joint capsule.

A Cobb elevator is then used to release the capsule medially and laterally, exposing the ankle joint. We recommend using the Cobb in the ankle joint to fully mobilize any adhesions within the ankle joint itself. Distraction of the ankle joint is then performed with either a pin distractor or lamina spreader. Preparation for arthrodesis is then performed with a series of curettes, osteotomy, or rotary burr. Emphasis is noted to debride the cartilaginous surfaces as well as the subchondral bone. We prefer to leave both the medial and lateral gutters unprepped for the potential for ankle arthrodesis take-down later in life. The subchondral bone is then drilled with a solid drill bit. This step is critical as it not only creates autologous bone graft but fragments the subchondral plate. An osteotome is then used to further fragment the subchondral plate.

Bone grafting is then used to increase the contact area, thus increasing the chance for arthrodesis. In most circumstances, cancellous grafting from the calcaneus provides an appropriate volume for isolated ankle arthrodesis. Occasionally, when significant bone voids exist, bulk structural allografts (autograft or allograft) may be considered. Orthobiologic supplementation may be considered based on patient

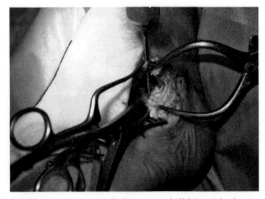

Fig. 29. Subchondral drilling using a small diameter drill bit with sleeve or fenestrating drill bit.

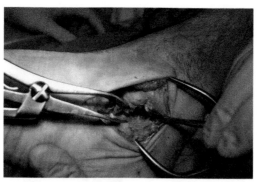

Fig. 30. "Fish scaling" the articular surfaces as a final step of joint preparation for arthrodesis.

comorbidities and surgeon discretion. The ankle joint is then reduced to neutral and pinned in place. When pinning the joint, most commonly a guidewire for the intended large cannulated screw is used. Either 1 or 2 wires can be placed. Care is taken to use a towel bump under the distal tibia to ensure appropriate reduction of the talar dome back into tibial plafond. Fluoroscopic examination is performed to ensure appropriate reduction and placement of the guidewire. In general, fluoroscopic evaluation should include appropriate reduction of frontal plane deformity, alignment of the lateral

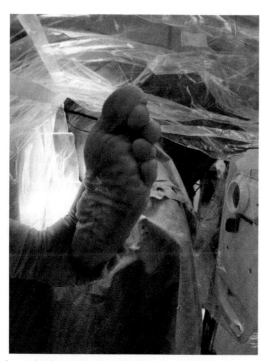

Fig. 31. Position the subtalar joint for fixation. Inversion of the valgus hindfoot to neutralize using the nondominant hand. A fluoroscopic image can be performed to check the reduction.

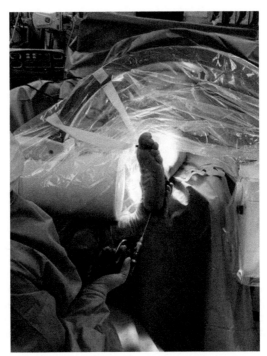

Fig. 32. Fluoroscopic imaging scout view obtained to confirm correct trajectory of guidewire for large diameter cannulated screw. A second guidewire may also be placed if 2 screw fixation is desired.

process of the middle of the tibial shaft on the lateral view, and neutral dorsiflexion. The first guidewire to be placed is the medial tibial face into the lateral process of the talus. When inserting this screw the talus will medialize and have intrinsic stability in the medial gutter. At this point the talus medialized and compression across the ankle joint, a secondary screw may be placed if desired. In general, we recommend using both crossed screws and an anterior plate to use additional construct stability via a tension band mechanism, when compared to anterior plating alone. An anterior ankle fusion plate is then placed and confirmed under fluoroscopic examination to be appropriately placed. Once confirmed the plate is pinned in place. The talar screws are initially placed securing the plate. If further compression is desired, eccentric drilling through the compression slots is performed. This will also ensure appropriate plate/bone contact. At this point, it is the surgeon's discretion to use either locking or nonlocking screw to complete the construct.

Closure is then performed in a layered fashion with emphasis on extensor retinaculum. The subcutaneous tissue is closed with either Vicryl or Monocryl. Skin closure is then performed by surgeon preference.

When deformity is present through the ankle joint, thorough preoperative planning must be performed. Congruent versus incongruent deformity needs to be fully examined. Intraarticular and extraarticular osteotomies may be created to help reduce the ankle joint to neutral. Typically, and intraarticular osteotomy will provide sufficient correction. We prefer to make the osteotomy within the distal tibia, creating a wedge-shaped resection.

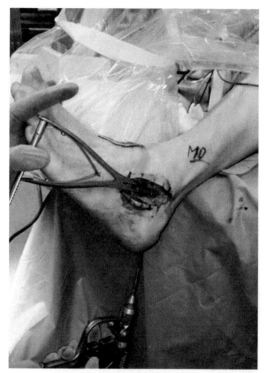

Fig. 33. Direct visualization of guidewire crossing central aspect of posterior facet. Lamina spreader is then removed, subtalar joint is positioned and guidewire is advanced into the talus.

Postop Protocol

Typical postoperative course will include a total of 5 to 6 weeks of non–weight-bearing immobilization. The first 1 to 2 weeks will be in a well-padded Robert Jones splint. At the first postoperative appointment, the patient will then be placed into a short leg non–weight-bearing cast. This is followed by 4 weeks in a removable cam walking boot. Pending radiographs, weight-bearing will be started. Physical therapy is initiated at 6-weeks postoperative. Transition back to regular shoe gear is typical around 10-weeks postoperative. We recommend the use of an ankle stabilizing orthosis during higher level activity such as running and jumping for an additional 4 weeks.

Complications

Some of the potential complications of the ankle arthrodesis include malunion, nonunion, hardware failure, hardware irritation, injury to the neurovascular bundle, adjacent joint arthritis, chronic gait change.

Pearls

- Straight anterior incision, which is placed in between the TA and EHL
- Tag suture placement on the extensor retinaculum for closure
- Retract the neurovascular bundle lateral during the dissection
- Refrain from excessive retraction
- Use of deep retraction (Gelpi retractor) if needed

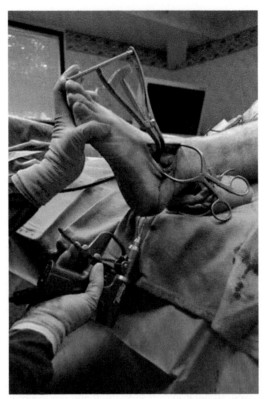

Fig. 34. An alternative view, the heel is suspended and stack of towels is placed under lower leg to facilitate positioning of the hindfoot while advancing the guidewire.

- Adequate joint preparation with appropriate joint fill with bone grafting
- Rigid fixation of the ankle joint
- Use of sagittal saw for deformity correction, if necessary

DISCUSSION

Mitchell and colleagues[23] noted that there was a reduction in revision rate as well as an increase in bony fusion with anterior ankle plating versus cannulated screws. This trend was further identified by Prissel and colleagues,[22] and furthermore, in that study, it was determined that the addition of the anterior plate did not alter the intended position of the fusion. Jeng and colleagues[21] noted that the order of screw placement is a personal choice. Medial, lateral, or posterior screws were equal with respect to pressure generated through the ankle joint. They further noted that the first screw achieves most of the compression. In general, we recommend using the first screw being from the medial tibia to the lateral talus as noted above. With this screw, we orient this screw slightly more vertical than the lateral screw so that the compressive force vector is relatively more vertical to maximize the compressive force at the interface of the tibial plafond and talar dome. Brodsky and colleagues[24] noted that patients who underwent ankle arthrodesis had a significant improvement ($P < .001$) in step length and velocity compared with their preoperative assessment.

In conclusion, anterior approach ankle arthrodesis provides a durable and predictable option for end-stage ankle arthritis. Although ankle arthroplasty is increasing in

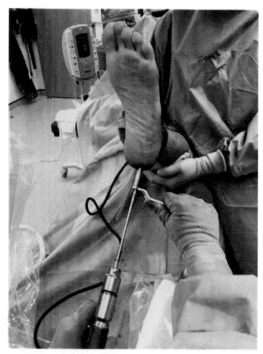

Fig. 35. Drill sleeve is used to protect soft tissues as drill is advanced just across talar articular surface.

utilization and percentage of successful outcomes at intermediate and long term, for some patients the better option remains arthrodesis.

Cases

#1. A 57-year-old woman presents 3 years following total ankle arthroplasty with continued pain. She has followed postoperative protocol as directed. The pain is progressively getting worst affecting her normal day-to-day activity. A full infection work up was performed resulting in negative blood work and cultures. A SPECT CT was performed showing increase uptake around both the tibial and talar components indicative of subsidence. A revision ankle arthroplasty versus ankle arthrodesis was discussed. She ultimately felt that ankle arthrodesis was a more appropriate option for her. A fresh femoral head was used as a bulk allograft. The calcar was used based on its strength. The cortical bone was fenestrated with a drill bit and DBM and rh-PDGF were placed around the outside. The bulk allograft was inserted into the deficit. Solid fixation was then placed spanning the graft and stabilizing the tibiotalar joint. Standard postoperative protocol was followed. The patient ultimately went onto mature fusion of the tibiotalar joint (**Figs. 38–47**).

#2. 61-year-old woman with uncontrolled diabetes mellitus, who previously underwent a cavus foot reconstruction and STJ arthrodesis. Unfortunately, following the STJ arthrodesis, she developed avascular necrosis of the lateral talar dome. In addition to diabetes mellitus, her medical history is complicated by severe lower back pain which required several corticosteroid injections and implantation of the spinal cord stimulator. She was offloaded in a patellar-bearing AFO for 18 months before definitive surgery for her ankle pain, allowing for improvement in her

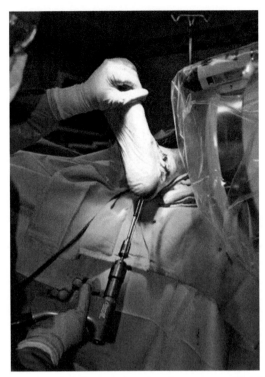

Fig. 36. Large diameter cannulated screw placed under power until at the level of the skin.

glycemic control and surgical management of her low back pain. Her ankle pain persisted despite the robust bracing attempt so she then proceeded with ankle arthrodesis via anterior approach with bulk allograft to the lateral talar dome and distal tibia. (**Figs. 48–52**)

TIBIOTALOCALCANEAL FUSION WITH NAIL
Introduction

Tibiotalocalcaneal (TTC) arthrodesis involves the fusion of the ankle and STJs to restore proper hindfoot alignment and remove painful arthritic joint motion. Fusion of both joints results in significant loss of hindfoot motion and functional deficit but can provide substantial pain relief and deformity correction. Most patients report favorable outcomes after undergoing TTC fusion nailing.[25] Utility of this extended arthrodesis has lessened with the advancement of TAR if realignment can be obtained. Still, TTC fusion remains useful in more severe deformities, high-demand patients, and as a salvage procedure.

Indications

Fusion of the ankle and the STJs is indicated in severe conditions after the failure of reasonable conservative measures. There are specific indications for TTC fusion. TTC fusion is indicated in severe hindfoot and ankle deformity with arthritic changes and loss of ligamentous support, such as stage 4 posterior tibialis tendon dysfunction.[26] This involves cases with irreducible hindfoot deformity and arthritis, with a valgus deformity of the ankle and deltoid ligament insufficiency. If the deltoid ligament

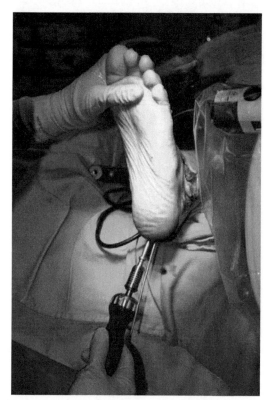

Fig. 37. Final screw insertion completed by hand.

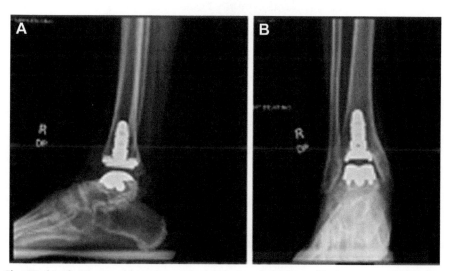

Fig. 38. (*A, B*): 57-year-old woman with a chronic pain in the ankle 3 years out from intramedullary total ankle arthroplasty.

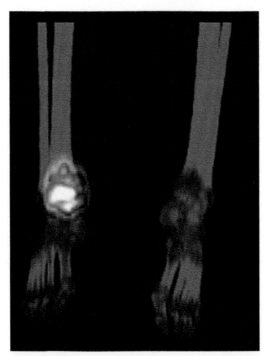

Fig. 39. SPECT CT indicating increased uptake in the tibial and talar components of the total ankle arthroplasty.

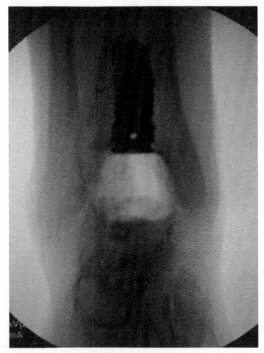

Fig. 40. Intraoperative radiograph demonstrating removal of the tibial tray and talar component of the total ankle arthroplasty.

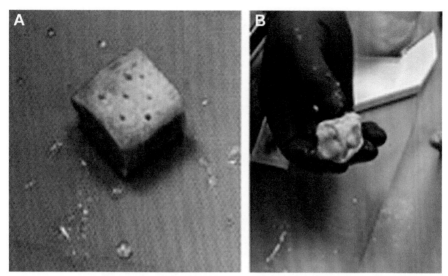

Fig. 41. (*A, B*): Preparation of femoral head bulk allograft for arthrodesis of the tibiotalar joint. Note the fenestrations through the cortical bone to encourage the incorporation of the graft. The graft is then coated with a mixture of demineralized bone matrix and r-PDGF.

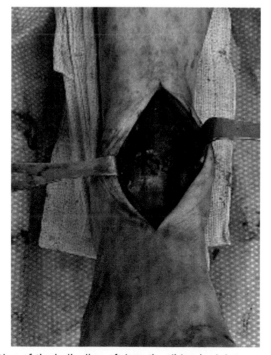

Fig. 42. Implantation of the bulk allograft into the tibiotalar joint.

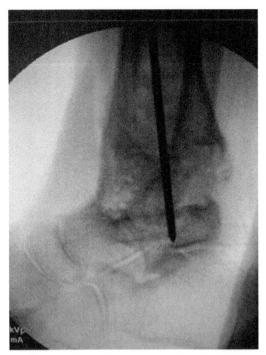

Fig. 43. Lateral radiograph with bulk allograft and guidewire for compression screw.

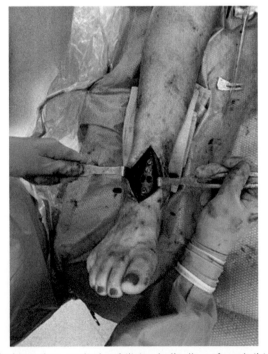

Fig. 44. Anterior locking plate applied stabilizing bulk allograft and tibiotalar joint.

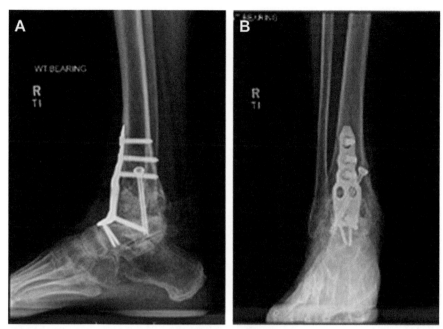

Fig. 45. (*A, B*): Postoperative radiographs demonstrating bone ingrowth into the bulk allograft and bone union of the tibiotalar joint.

cannot be reconstructed, TAR should not be undertaken, and thus fusion may be a better option. Revision fusion with a TTC construct is indicated in cases of previous failed fusion attempts resulting in malunion or nonunion.[27] TTC fusion can also be done after the failure of TAR, even in the face of substantial bone loss at the fusion site.[28]

TTC fusion can be achieved with external fixation, plates, screws, and intramedullary nail constructs. The intramedullary nail technique has the benefit of load sharing which allows additional compression across the fusion surface and the ability to be performed through smaller dissection than plating. Lack of adequate blood supply from previous trauma or avascular necrosis of the talar body may benefit from extended fusion and load-sharing properties of the intramedullary nail.[29] The load-sharing property has also proved useful in the poor bone stock and loss of structure seen in Charcot neuroarthropathy of the ankle and hindfoot.[30] The combined arthrodesis of the ankle and STJ has been useful as both a primary and salvage procedure in cases of severe deformity and arthritis not amenable to ankle joint replacement.

Complications and Risk Factors

Complications after TTC fusion nailing include infection, nerve damage, delayed wound healing, hardware failure, malunion, and nonunion. The nonunion rate after TTC nailing has been reported to be around 17% for the subalar joint and 9% for the ankle joint, with not all of these patients being symptomatic.[31] Risk factors for nonunion with TTC nailing include diabetes with Hgb A1c > 7.5, diabetic neuropathy, American Society of Anesthesiologists (ASA) score greater than 2, and Charcot neuroarthropathy.[32] A 2021 systematic review by Patel and colleagues[33] found preexisting peripheral neuropathy as the risk factor most associated with nonunion after TTC

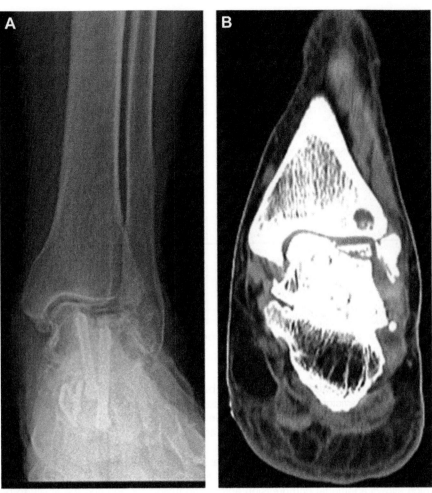

Fig. 46. (A, B): Radiographic and CT imaging of a large lateral talus osteochondral defect with underlying tibial cyst.

nailing. Patient selection can help to mitigate these risks and inform patients about potential negative outcomes including the need for revision surgery or amputation.

Technique

A long (15–20 cm) lateral incision is placed over the fibula extending over the sinus tarsi, and a 5 to 7 cm anteromedial ankle gutter incision is used for the medial ankle joint. This allows for fibular osteotomy and graft harvest, excellent exposure to the ankle joint and STJ, and facilitates any deformity correction that may be needed. The medial incision can be used to prepare the medial ankle joint, but also to allow for the medialization of the talus. Dissection is carried deep to the fibula, with care being taken to avoid damage to the sural nerve and peroneal tendons. The anterior and distal aspect of the fibula is freed of all soft tissue attachments, and the level of fibular osteotomy is determined. In this case, an oblique osteotomy is made, and a second osteotomy is made approximately 1 cm proximal. A section of bone is removed to

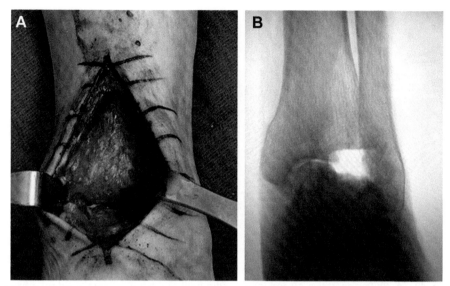

Fig. 47. (*A, B*): Intraoperative imaging demonstrating resection arthroplasty of the talus and distal tibia.

allow for shortening. The fibula is then freed medially of the syndesmotic attachments and rotated laterally. The medial half of the fibula is then resected using a sagittal saw, with the medial side removed for bone graft and the lateral half left with the posterior attachments intact (**Fig. 53**). This allows for the exposure of the ankle and STJs. The medial incision is then deepened to the ankle and an arthrotomy is performed to allow access to the medial ankle joint.

Joint preparation is performed in a typical fashion with distraction of the ankle and STJ, removal of the articular cartilage and subchondral bone, followed by fenestration and fish-scaling (**Fig. 54**). While curettage is preferred, in the case of severe deformity, planar resection of the ankle joint with a sagittal saw may be used. Attention is directed

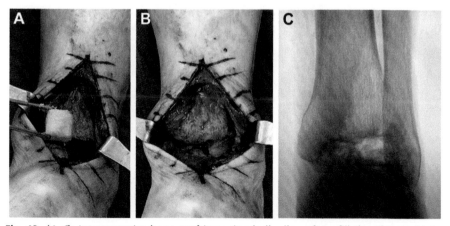

Fig. 48. (*A–C*): Intraoperative bone grafting using bulk allograft to fill the tibia and talus deficit.

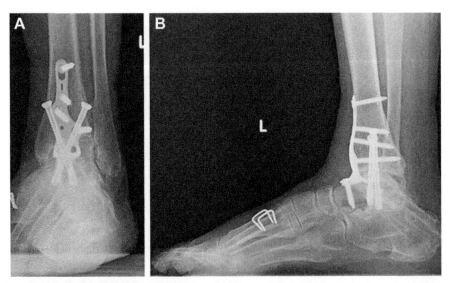

Fig. 49. (A, B): Postoperative AP and lateral radiographs with bulk allograft and solid fixation with locking plate.

to the medial ankle joint to ensure full joint preparation. The medial talus and lateral side of the medial malleolus can be resected to allow for the medialization of the talus under the tibia if needed.

After thorough resection of the joints, the ankle and hindfoot are typically very loose. Careful positioning of the ankle and hindfoot are undertaken. A line is drawn along the tibial crest and along the 2nd metatarsal shaft. This will help visualize internal and external rotation. Once the joints are prepared for fusion, a guidewire is placed from the calcaneus into the tibia. This must be done with the foot and ankle held in proper alignment. The wire is then checked with AP, lateral, and axial intraoperative images.

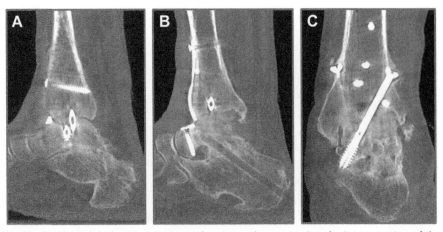

Fig. 50. (A–C). Weight-bearing CT 4-months postop demonstrating the incorporation of the allograft with osseous fusion. *Tibiotalocalcaneal fusion with nail.*

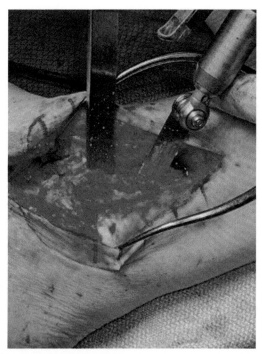

Fig. 51. A lateral clinical image of the fibula after initial dissection. The anterior and distal soft tissues are stripped off the fibula. Then, a sagittal saw is used to split the fibula into medial and lateral sections. The medial half is harvested and used as morselized bone graft. The lateral half is retracted out of the way and later used as onlay bone graft to support the lateral ankle and preserve a fibular remnant.

All these images are necessary as the wire can be missed in several directions and must be confirmed. If the position of the foot is inadequate, the wire is removed, the foot is repositioned, and the wire is redriven. A plantar incision is made around the wire, and an entry drill is advanced from the calcaneus to the tibia. Then reaming is done in a sequential fashion. The goal is to feel cortical chatter, indicating a good fill of the canal, and to extend more proximally than the anticipated nail length. The nail is usually then sized 1 to 1.5 mm under the reaming diameter. The reaming from the canal will act as bone graft in the fusion sight. The intramedullary nail can be placed with the manufacturer's guidelines, compressed and interlocking screws placed. Once the nail is placed, the fibular onlay graft is placed. It is rotated via the posterior attachments back into position lateral along the tibia, talus, and calcaneus. Once in position, the fibula can be secured with either 4.0 to 5.0 mm cannulated screws or the interlocking screws for the nail.

Case Example

A 47-year-old man with progressive angular deformity of his ankle presented after having failed a custom brace. Radiographs showed significant ankle deformity and hindfoot arthritis (**Fig. 55**). Computed tomography confirmed a 25° varus deformity at the ankle joint and significant syndesmotic injury. Options including TAR were presented. TTC arthrodesis was pursued due to activity in manual labor, progressive nature of the deformity, and age. Fibula onlay graft was performed as well.

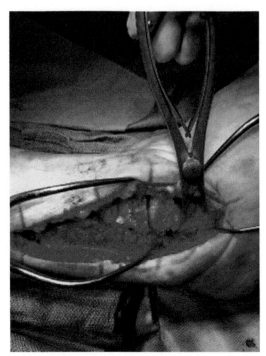

Fig. 52. A lateral clinical image showing the lateral half of the fibula retracted posteriorly, and the ankle and subtalar joints exposed and prepared.

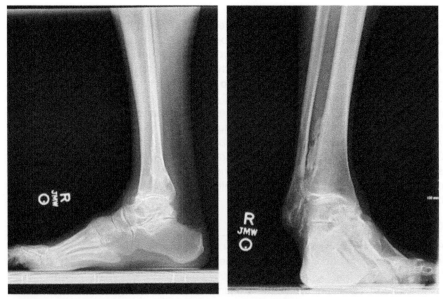

Fig. 53. Lateral and AP radiographs of an ankle and hindfoot insignificant incongruent ankle varus and subtalar joint arthritis.

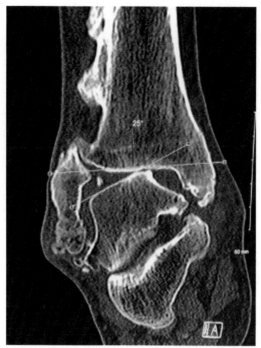

Fig. 54. Coronal plane CT scan demonstrating 25° incongruent varus with loose body formation, lateral impingement, and subtalar arthritis.

Pearls

- Ensure the talus is medialized. Otherwise, bisection of the calcaneus is lateral to central tibia and is then off axis
- Use of a stack of towels behind the foot and ankle to aid in the alignment of the tibiotalar joint
- When performing the first fibular osteotomy, a second osteotomy made proximally to remove 1 cm of bone will help with any shortening that will occur from fusion at the ankle and STJs.
- Through the anteromedial incision, a deltoid release will help to mobilize the joint to facilitate the medial joint preparation as well as positioning.
- A 7″ Gelpi retractor is used laterally between the anterior soft tissue and remaining lateral fibula to ensure exposure to the ankle and STJs, but keeping the posterior fibular attachments
- When using an intramedullary nail, after placing the first guidewire, often the foot and ankle are positioned correctly, but the wire may be off. Leave the 1st wire as a stabilizer and guide and place a second wire in the proper position.
- When using an intramedullary nail, check to make sure that the posterior to anterior calcaneal screw is in the right alignment before any other screws are placed. Poor rotation of the nail may cause this screw to skive the medial or lateral wall of the calcaneus making placement difficult.
- If additional bone graft is needed for the arthrodesis, a Reamer-Irrigator-Aspirator may be used to ream up to the proximal tibia to obtain autogenous graft.

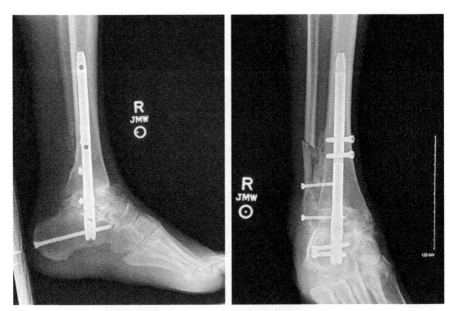

Fig. 55. Ap and lateral radiographs after tibiotalocalcaneal arthrodesis with intramedullary nail and lateral fibular onlay graft. Excellent correction and compression of the joints is noted.

DISCLOSURE: (RELEVANT DISCLOSURES LISTED)

R.T. Scott – Medline, Stryker, Wright Medical, M. Dujela - None, J.G. DeVries – Nextremity, Carbofix, C. Hyer – Wright Medical, Stryker, M. Prissel – Medline, NovaStep, Paragon 28, T. Langan – Medline, B. Van Dyke - Medline.

REFERENCES

1. Gilgen A, Knupp M, Hintermann B. Subtalar and naviculocuneiform arthrodesis for the treatment of hindfoot valgus with collapse of the medial arch. Tech Foot Ankle Surg 2013;12(4):190–5.

2. Gerrity M, Williams M. Naviculocuneiform arthrodesis in adult flatfoot: a case series. J Foot Ankle Surg 2019;58(2):352–6.

3. Budny AM, Grossman JP. Naviculocuneiform arthrodesis. Clin Podiatr Med Surg 2007;24(4):753–63.

4. Ajis A, Geary N. Surgical technique, fusion rates, and planovalgus foot deformity correction with naviculocuneiform fusion. Foot Ankle Int 2014;35(3):232–7.

5. Steiner CS, Gilgen A, Zwicky L, et al. Combined subtalar and naviculocuneiform fusion for treating adult acquired flatfoot deformity with medial arch collapse at the level of the naviculocuneiform joint. Foot Ankle Int 2019;40(1):42–7.

6. Hyer CF, Galli MM, Scott RT, et al. Ankle valgus after hindfoot arthrodesis: a radiographic and chart comparison of the medial double and triple arthrodeses. J Foot Ankle Surg 2014;53(1):55–8.

7. DeVries JG, Scharer B. Hindfoot deformity corrected with double versus triple arthrodesis: radiographic comparison. J Foot Ankle Surg 2015;54(3):424–7.

8. Berlet GC, Hyer CF, Scott RT, et al. Medial double arthrodesis with lateral column sparing and arthrodiastasis: a radiographic and medical record review. J Foot Ankle Surg 2015;54(3):441–4.

9. Vora Anand M, Myerson Mark S, Jeng Clifford L. The medial approach to triple arthrodesis: indications and technique for management of rigid valgus deformities in high-risk patients. Tech Foot Ankle Surg 2005;44:258–62.

10. Jeng CL, Tankson CJ, Myerson MS. The single medial approach to triple arthrodesis: a cadaver study. Foot Ankle Int 2006;27(12):1022–5.

11. Jackson WFM, Tryfonidis M, Cooke PH, et al. Arthrodesis of the hindfoot for valgus deformity: an entirely medial approach. J bone Jt Surg Br volume 2007; 89(7):925–7.

12. De Wachter J, Knupp M, Beat H. Double-hindfoot arthrodesis through a single medial approach. Tech Foot Ankle Surg 2007;6(4):237–42.

13. Coetzee JC, Hansen ST. Surgical management of severe deformity resulting from posterior tibial tendon dysfunction. Foot Ankle Int 2001;22(12):944–9.

14. Galli, M. M., Scott, R. T., Bussewitz, B., et al (2014). Structures at risk with medial double hindfoot fusion: a cadaveric study. J Foot Ankle Surg, 53(5), 598.

15. Kulik S, Clanton T. Tarsal coalition. Foot Ankle Int 1996;17(5):286–96.

16. Carr J, Hansen S, Bernirschke SK. Subtalar distraction bone block fusion for late complications of os calcis fractures. Foot Ankle 1998;9(2):81–9.

17. Diezi C, Favre P, Vienne P. Primary isolated subtalar arthrodesis: outcomes after 2-5 years followup. Foot Ankle Int 2008;29(12):111–95 -1202.

18. Fornaciari P, Gilgen A, Zwicky L, et al. Isolated talonavicular fusion with tension band for Muller-Weiss syndrome. Foot Ankle Int 2014;35(12):1316–22.

19. Fortin PT. Posterior tibial tendon insufficiency. Isolated fusion of the talonavicular joint. Foot Ankle Clin 2001;6(1):137–51.

20. Astion DJ, Deland JT, Otis JC, et al. Motion of the hindfoot after simulated arthrodesis. J Bone Joint Surg Am 1997;79(2):241–6.

21. Jeng CL, Baumbach SF, Campbell J, et al. Comparison of initial compression of the medial, lateral, and posterior screws in an ankle fusion construct. Foot Ankle Int 2011;32(1):71–6.

22. Prissel MA, Simpson GA, Sutphen SA, et al. Ankle Arthrodesis: a retrospective analysis comparing single column, locked anterior plating to crossed lag screw technique. J Foot Ankle Surg 2017;56(3):453–6.

23. Mitchell PM, Douleh DG, Thomson B. Comparison of ankle fusion rates with and without anterior plate augmentation. Foot Aankle Int 2016;38(4):419–23.

24. Brodsky JW, Kane JM, Coleman J, et al. Abnormalities of gait caused by ankle arthritis are improved by ankle arthrodesis. J Bone Joint Surg 2016;98-B: 1369–75.

25. Ajis A, Tan KJ, Myerson MS. Ankle arthrodesis vs TTC arthrodesis: patient outcomes, satisfaction and return to activity. Foot Ankle Int 2013;34(5):657–65.

26. Myerson MS. Adult acquired flatfoot deformity: treatment of dysfunction of the posterior tibial tendon. J Bone Joint Surg Am 1996;78-A:780–92.

27. DeVries JG, Nguyen M, Berlet GC, et al. The effect of recombinant bone morphogenetic protein-2 in revision tibiotalocalcaneal arthrodesis: utilization of the retrograde arthrodesis intramedullary nail database. J Foot Ankle Surg 2012;51: 426–32.

28. Bussewitz B, DeVries JG, Dujela M, et al. Retrograde intramedullary nail with femoral head allograft for large deficit tibiotalocalcaneal arthrodesis. Foot Ankle Int 2014;35:706–11.

29. DeVries JG, Philbin TM, Hyer CF. Retrograde intramedullary nail arthrodesis for avascular necrosis of the talus. Foot Ankle Int 2010;31(11):965–72.

30. DeVries JG, Berlet GC, Hyer CF. A retrospective comparative analysis of Charcot ankle stabilization using an intramedullary rod with or without application of circular external fixator – utilization of the retrograde arthrodesis intramedullary nail database. J Foot Ankle Surg 2012;51:420–5.

31. Dujela M, Hyer C, Berlet G. Rate of subtalar joint arthrodesis after retrograde tibiotalocalcaneal arthrodesis with intramedullary nail fixation: evelution of RAIN Database. Foot Ankle Spec 2018;11:410–5.

32. Kowalski C, Stauch C, Callahan R, et al. Prognostic risk factors for complications associated with tibiotalocalcaneal arthrodesis with a nail. Foot Ankle Surg 2020; 26:708–11.

33. Patel S, Baker L, Perez J, et al. Risk factors for nonunion following tibiotalocalcaneal arthrodesis: a systematic review and meta-analysis. Foot Ankle Surg 2021. https://doi.org/10.1016/j.fas.2021.02.010.

Current Techniques in Total Ankle Arthroplasty

James M. Cottom, DPM, FACFAS[a],*, Jason George DeVries, DPM, FACFAS[b],
Christopher F. Hyer, DPM, MS, FACFAS[c], Jeffrey E. McAlister, DPM, FACFAS[d],
Matthew D. Sorensen, DPM, FACFAS[e]

KEYWORDS

- Ankle arthritis • Ankle replacement • Total ankle arthroplasty • Valgus ankle
- Varus ankle

KEY POINTS

- Proper patient selection is paramount for a successful outcome in total ankle replacement.
- Deformities above and below the ankle joint must be addressed properly for a favorable long-term outcome.
- When coronal plane deformities are present either a single or staged approach should be considered based on the amount of deformity, whereby it is originating from and surgeon experience.
- Patients should extensively be consulted before undergoing a total ankle on risks, complications as well as outcomes and the possibility for additional procedures if failure occurs.

INTRODUCTION

Total ankle replacement (TAR) continues to increase in popularity as a motion-preserving option to ankle arthrodesis. TAR is indicated for primary, posttraumatic, and inflammatory arthropathies as an alternative procedure to tibiotalar arthrodesis. Proper patient selection is paramount to a successful outcome in TAR. Contraindications to TAR include the presence of neuropathy, active infection, severe peripheral arterial disease, inadequate bone stock, and severe uncorrectable coronal plane deformity.[1] This article is a brief overview of techniques and PEARLS on how to address a well-aligned ankle joint, varus deformity as well as valgus deformities as well as the authors experience with single versus staging coronal plane deformities.

[a] Florida Orthopedic Foot & Ankle Center, 1630 S. Tuttle Avenue, Sarasota, FL 34239, USA;
[b] Orthopedics & Sports Medicine - BayCare Clinic, 501 N. 10th Street, Manitowoc, WI 54220, USA; [c] Orthopedic Foot & Ankle Center, 350 W. Wilson Bridge Road, Worthington, OH 43085, USA; [d] Phoenix Foot and Ankle Institute, 7301 E 2nd Street, Ste 206, Scottsdale, AZ 85251, USA; [e] Weil Foot & Ankle Institute, 1900 Hollister Dr., Suite 160, Libertyville, IL 60048, USA
* Corresponding author.
E-mail address: drcottom@flofac.com

Clin Podiatr Med Surg 39 (2022) 273–293
https://doi.org/10.1016/j.cpm.2021.11.012
0891-8422/22/© 2021 Elsevier Inc. All rights reserved.

PRIMARY, NEUTRAL TOTAL ANKLE REPLACEMENT

While TAR continues to expand and be used in more complicated cases[2] primary surgery in neutrally aligned ankles will continue to be needed. This is often recommended to newer foot and ankle surgeons as the types of cases that should be attempted first in practice as there is a learning curve.[3,4] Even in the case of experienced surgeons, with the continued advent of new systems, prudence may dictate that new implants be first used in an uncomplicated ankle.

The goals of any ankle replacement include pain relief and function restoration. In the case of a primary, neutrally aligned ankle, several other goals can also be achieved. *Bone preservation* should be considered to maintain as much as the patient's own anatomy as the ankle allows. This is important especially in a neutrally aligned ankle as the joint itself is should not require large bone cuts to correct for deformity. The preservation of the dense subchondral bone has also been suggested to be helpful as support for a metallic prosthesis. It can also help prepare for potential long-term issues. While implants have shown good midterm results at 7 to 12 years with success rates more than 90%,[5–7] potential need for more surgery or even formal revisions is possible after TAR. *Motion preservation or restoration* should be considered as well. The best predictor of motion after TAR is usually the motion preoperatively, but restoration of motion is possible.[8] This will allow for the protection of the adjacent joints and prevent future hindfoot fusions.[9] Care taken to not over stuff the joint may allow for good motion afterward, and minimal incisions to prevent excessive scar and fibrosis is helpful.

When referring to the "neutral" ankle, this refers to more than simply the coronal plane deformity, although this is certainly a primary factor. When discussing neutral alignment, this is referring to deformity of less than 10° of varus or valgus.[10,11] While this is not perfectly neutral by definition, it is also something that can usually be corrected with minimal intervention, minimal change in operative procedure, and should not add significant time to the Case. Soft tissue releases, especially deltoid ligament releases and Broström lateral ankle ligament repairs may be undertaken, even in the neutral ankle. It does mean that the ankle must have a degree of inherent balance and not require more advanced or complicated soft tissue repair or ligament reconstruction. In addition to the coronal plane, the sagittal and transverse planes must be either aligned or easily corrected. An ankle that is in plantarflexion may still be considered neutral if it can be corrected with joint decompression, polyethylene spacer size, and posterior muscle group deformity. Anterior and posterior translation is often encountered and again is still considered "neutral" in most cases. If the translation can be corrected with soft tissue release or by using a fixed or a biased polyethylene spacer no major deviation of the technique is needed.

When referring to the "primary" ankle, certainly this refers to cases in which a total ankle has not been previously performed. This also requires that no previous ankle arthrodesis has been attempted as that can dramatically change the soft tissue excursion, incision placement, and bony anatomy. Besides these obvious definitions of "primary" in the case of TAR, several other factors may be considered when treating an arthritic ankle as "primary." Previous ankle trauma, even previous fracture and fixation can still be considered a primary replacement. Indeed, most ankle arthritis is posttraumatic.[12,13] However, in cases in which there is poor bone stock, adjacent hindfoot arthritis requiring arthrodesis, and extensive hardware present there may need to be adjustments made that are above what a "primary" ankle should require. These additional concerns can come from systemic disease such as rheumatoid arthritis or more extensive and involved previous trauma and should not be approached without appropriately planning.

Technique

The technique for primary, neutral TAR can be approached without deviations needed to accommodate extenuating circumstances or additional procedures. Meticulous attention to bone and motion preservation and prevention of wound or neurovascular complications is paramount. The incision is made longitudinally over the ankle lateral to the tibialis anterior (TA). No retraction of the skin and soft tissue should be used in the superficial layers. Dissection is carried to the extensor retinaculum which is sharply incised and tagged for later repair. Deep to this layer are the tendon sheaths for the TA, extensor hallucis longus (EHL), and extensor digitorum longus (EDL) tendons. An interval lateral to the TA is made with care being made to keep the tendon in its sheath. The neurovascular bundle is then identified and retracted. At this point deep retraction can be performed and the anterior ankle joint is encountered and opened in a longitudinal direction. The capsular and periosteal tissues are elevated sharply and with the use of a Cobb elevator. A Gelpi self-retaining retractor can now be placed in this deep capsular layer. Dissection proximally and distally is taken only to the extent that alignment can be seen, and any jigs can be placed. While not a minimally invasive procedure, in the Case of primary, straightforward ankle replacement, excessive dissection is to be avoided.

Once the joint is opened, different ankle implants will have different specific steps to perform. However, several consistent steps are undertaken. Soft tissue releases are performed as needed before bony cuts. This often includes simple releases of the medial or lateral ligaments. Even in the case of a truly neutral ankle, long-term scarring, arthritis, and immobility needs to be addressed and release of any fibrotic structures is helpful (**Fig. 1**). The tibial and talar cuts are made and the bone segments removed. This can be done en bloc or piece meal depending on the anatomy and patient. However, in the case or primary and well-aligned ankles, bone preservation again is important. After the bone resection is done, the posterior capsule is assessed. At minimum there needs to be a thorough flush of this area to remove bone debris from the cuts, and in more rigid cases resection of the capsule is performed. Either way the goal is to allow for more motion, initially by removing any contracture or fibrosis, and long term by minimizing risk of heterotopic ossification.

The components are placed according to the specific implant being used. Again, coronal plane placement is important, but so is anterior to posterior position as well as rotation. After implantation of the components, the ankle is run through range of motion to assess for any deficiencies. Mild deltoid or lateral ligament instability may

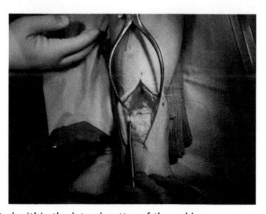

Fig. 1. Fibrosis noted within the lateral gutter of the ankle.

be corrected with increasing the polyethylene thickness. Conversely, repair or tightening of the lateral ligaments has been shown to be helpful. A deficiency in dorsiflexion is addressed with posterior muscle group lengthening, typically a gastrocnemius recession. Final images, including dorsiflexion and plantarflexion images are taken. A layer closure is performed, with meticulous attention paid to the extensor retinaculum. Protection of the anterior ankle and the TA tendon is crucial for success.

Case

55-year-old woman with previous osteochondral defect treatment with arthroscopy and microfracture. While she did well initially, pain recurred over time. Radiographs showed a medial talus osteochondral defect (**Fig. 2**). MRI was ordered to assess the recurrent lesion more fully, and was shown to be a 2 × 2 cm recurrent medial osteochondral defect, with associated tibial injury (**Fig. 3**). Options discussed included revision arthroscopy, fusion, or replacement. CT scan was obtained and confirmed a large, shallow medial osteochondral defect (**Fig. 4**). A low profile tibial and talus resurfacing implant was chosen to preserve bone. Range of motion was assessed, and a gastrocnemius recession was performed (**Fig. 5**). At 1 year out from surgery patient is functioning well with good component incorporation (**Fig. 6**).

VARUS ANKLE

Angular deformity in the coronal plane is a difficult and challenging Case that requires special attention to all 3 planes to accomplish the desired goals.

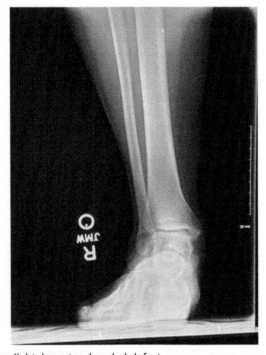

Fig. 2. Note the medial talus osteochondral defect.

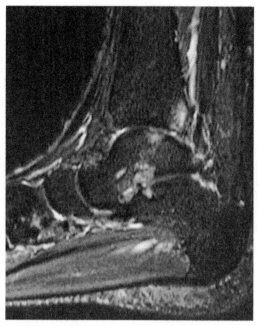

Fig. 3. MRI demonstrating the defect in the talus and tibia.

Patients specifically in varus tend to have a classic presentation and symptoms that should be discussed. Long-standing hindfoot varus deformities and a compensated forefoot valgus can present with thickened hyperkeratotic lesions on the plantar lateral aspect of the heel, the fifth metatarsal base and often the fifth metatarsal head. These

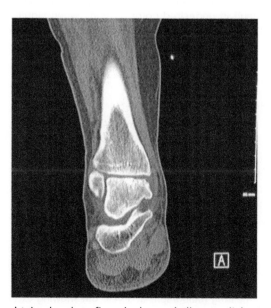

Fig. 4. CT scan was obtained and confirmed a large, shallow medial osteochondral defect.

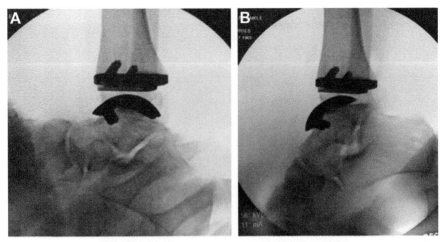

Fig. 5. (A, B) A low profile tibial and talus resurfacing implant was chosen to preserve bone.

can be presenting complaints that often require a higher level of attention and radiographs that one would often not consider. There is a reason why the patient has the lesions and often times a deformity from lateral ankle instability or previous trauma to the lateral ligament complex can be uncovered through a complete history and physical. Often patients have lateral foot pain and medial ankle gutter pain which can translate up into the tibial spine. This can be misconstrued as posterior tibial tendinitis. A very thorough lateral ankle physical examination should be performed as well as a gait assessment/analysis. Above and beyond the word limit of this section is a cavus foot reconstruction review but please take it into consideration.

Varus deformities are typically discussed as staged or primary procedures when the deformity is at the ankle, and we aren't discussing ankle arthrodesis. Ankle arthroplasty can result in undesired complications when significant coronal plane deformity of the foot and/or ankle is present, and the complexity of the case is challenging.[14–16]

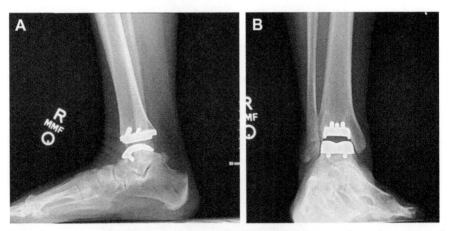

Fig. 6. (A, B) Weight-bearing radiographs at 1 year out showing excellent alignment and bone ingrowth.

PRIMARY VARUS CORRECTION

Ankle arthroplasty can be accomplished in a primary deformity correction Case, whereby the ankle deformity is corrected with the use of cut guides and no significant foot correction is needed. This is often the case when the ankle deformity is congruent or less than 10° of deformity. The center of rotation of angulation (CORA) needs to be determined as well and most often it is at the level of the ankle. These cases are usually easier to correct with the utility of cut guides because the deformity is within the ankle and the deltoid is still competent (unlike incongruent ankle varus). The context of this particular section is not to persuade the reader to use a semiconstrained or mobile device, but to make recommendations based on authors' experience with these complex deformities. Preoperative standard ankle and foot radiographs are reviewed along with a long leg axial or calcaneal axial to appreciate the degree of hindfoot varus deformity. This can significantly help with surgical efficiencies and patient outcomes. Assessing not only ankle arthritic changes but any hindfoot arthritic changes or previous trauma or surgical procedures.

A common situation that may present is a congruent varus deformity of the ankle with significant arthroses in the medial gutter, a positive talar tilt and/or talar tilt, and no obvious intrinsic calcaneal varum (**Fig. 7**). Sequentially, the order of operation is proximal to distal with the plan and consent focused deformity correction of the ankle and related ancillary procedures. There are situations whereby a medial opening tibial wedge osteotomy may be performed but often the deformity can be "cut out" without the significant comorbidity of the tibial osteotomy.

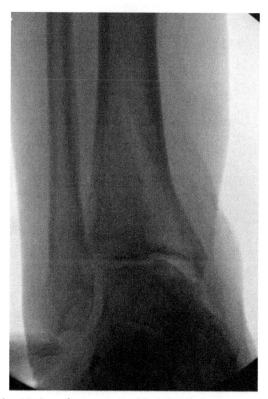

Fig. 7. Intraoperative AP view of congruent ankle deformity with medial malleolar collapse.

Key components to primary congruent ankle varus deformity can be visualized initially when the mortise view is examined after the ankle arthroplasty system is applied. The authors recommend correcting the posterior muscle group tightness first as necessary. Next, as seen in **Fig. 8**, the ankle arthroplasty system can be applied perpendicular to the anatomic/mechanical axis of the limb. Do not focus on the talus at this point, just the tibia. Here the fibula is used as a fulcrum on which the lateral process of the talus is pushed down after the tibia is cut. Once the tibia is cut with the surgeon's preferred arthroplasty system and the tibia is removed, the deltoid ligament peel is performed with a Cobb elevator releasing as much of the deltoid ligament as possible. The goal here is to get the talus as flat or perpendicular to the tibial cut as possible. One has to be careful not to make the tibial cut too high which can lead to unwanted tibial fractures. This can be accomplished by pulling or pushing the talus down with a lamina spreader, pin-to-pin spreader or simply manual control of the heel (**Fig. 9**).

If this cannot be accomplished, which is uncommon, then a medial malleolar osteotomy can be performed from an anterior approach with a small sagittal saw below the level of the tibial cut. The talus is allowed to relax or fall out of a varus position which essentially lengthens the deltoid ligaments. The gap is then filled with bone from the tibial cut. The osteotomy can be fixated with surgeon's preference of screws and

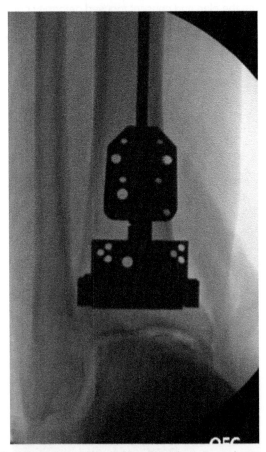

Fig. 8. Intraoperative application of the ankle arthroplasty jig and cut guide which show a tibial cut that is neutral to the long axis of the leg.

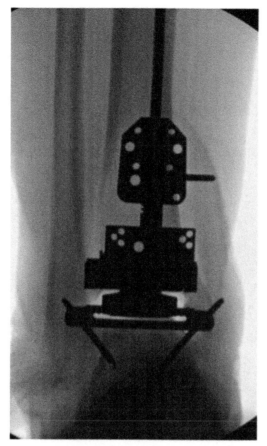

Fig. 9. Manual reduction of the deformity and pinning the talus in the desired position allows for optimal talar dome preparation.

plates. Often this can easily be performed in a revision Case or if there are positive inversion stress tests (**Figs. 10–13**).

Next, after the talar cut is performed with the talus in a neutral position in all planes, the implants may be inserted. Typically, a thicker polyethylene may be necessary due to an increased amount of tibial resection but is certainly case dependent. **Figs. 14** and **15** show final constructs after varus correction.

Finally, as with any ankle arthroplasty case the integrity of the ankle ligaments is tested under fluoroscopy and the foot posture (heel varus and any forefoot deformity) are confirmed to be neutral. When the CORA is at the ankle, and especially when these cases are congruent, usually the only secondary procedure that is necessary is a lateral ankle reconstruction (Brostrom or Brostrom-Evans). The authors recommend keeping ancillary procedures to a minimum during primary ankle arthroplasty procedures to reduce complications.

STAGED VARUS CORRECTION

These are even more challenging than previously mentioned due to extrinsic factors outside of the ankle joint itself. When a patient presents with over 10 to 15° of ankle

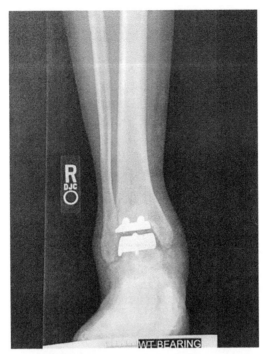

Fig. 10. Weightbearing AP image of a varus ankle arthroplasty which was painful medially and lacked adequate range of motion.

incongruent varus, one should safely assume that the lateral ligaments and peroneal tendons have been incompetent for some time. These are patients in whom the authors recommend staging. Often times chronic ankle instability or peroneal weakness can drive the ankle into varus which is then compounded by a calcaneal varus and midfoot contracture. When the peroneal tendons, specifically the peroneus brevis become disengaged or torn, then the posterior tibial tendon and peroneus longus become unopposed which will drive pain in the fifth metatarsal base and medial ankle compartment. This is why a thorough examination of the peroneals is important in the patient's outcome and helps identify whether or not these should be done in a staged fashion. If the authors suspect significant weakness of the peroneals, the preoperative workup will include an MRI. Preparing the patient for a staged procedure is important and reviewing the expectations and healing process. If a staged procedure is planned, the authors' recommendation of at least 3 to 6 weeks between the procedures to allow for soft tissue healing to occur (eg,. peroneal tendon repair or allograft reconstruction or calcaneal osteotomy).

In a staged approach, the authors' primary goal is to allow healing of the soft tissues and get the ankle in neutral for the ankle arthroplasty. This makes for a very smooth and efficient implantation process, minimizes tourniquet time, reduces coagulopathy concerns, and will decrease the time the implant will be stationary.

Figs. 16 and **17** show an incongruent ankle varus in a patient with a previous simple Brostrom and medial malleolar arthrosis. Preoperative MRI showed severe peroneal tendinopathy and manual muscle testing was confirmatory. The same approach as previously described is utilized here with a proximal to distal approach (**Fig. 18**). A

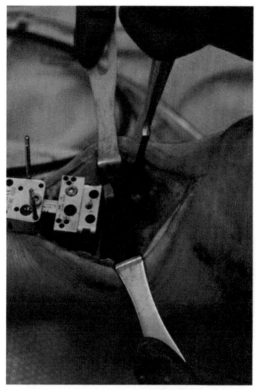

Fig. 11. Intraoperative view of a medial malleolar osteotomy which allowed for the lengthening of the deltoid and reduction in varus deformity correction after the tibia was recut.

lateral calcaneal wedge osteotomy is performed to mitigate any varus pull of the posterior muscle group. Then, the peroneal tendons and lateral ankle ligament complex is repaired as necessary with allograft reconstruction or tendon transfer. The lateral ligaments are then repaired as desired, seen here with a Brostrom-Evans, using a deficient peroneus brevis (**Fig. 19**). Next, a small anterior incision can be performed, and cement inserted in the medial gutter and or pinned in a neutral position (**Figs. 20** and

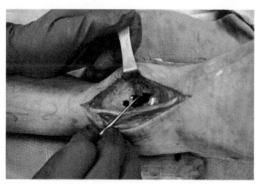

Fig. 12. Calcaneal autograft seen here being inserted to the resting position, if not slightly opened, of the medial malleolus and deltoid ligament.

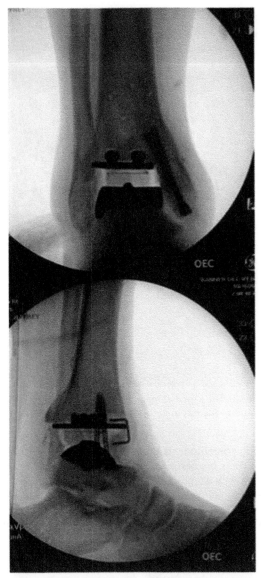

Fig. 13. The final AP and lateral intraoperative radiographs of a revision ankle arthroplasty after the tibial cut was adjusted and the medial malleolar osteotomy was fixated.

21). This trend is to allow the deltoids to stretch out and be released before the arthroplasty is performed. As stated in the previous section, a stress inversion test and anterior drawer is performed to confirm stability of the ankle before pinning.

The second stage, as described previously, is performed 3 to 6 weeks later. The cement is removed, the stabilizing wires are removed, and the ankle arthroplasty inserted. Here the authors do lean toward recommending a semiconstrained or fixed component device (**Figs. 22** and **23**). This time delay allows less vascular stress on the anterior incision among other advantages.

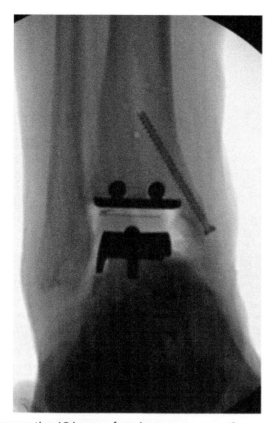

Fig. 14. Final intraoperative AP image of a primary varus correction.

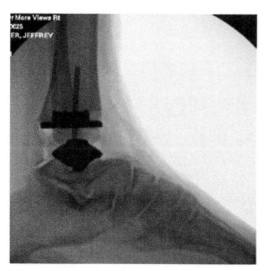

Fig. 15. Final lateral fluoroscopic image of a primary varus correction after Brostrom was performed.

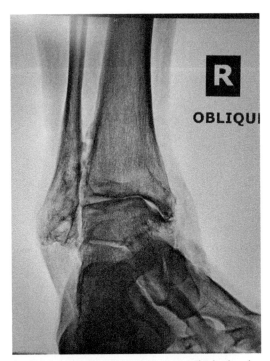

Fig. 16. Weightbearing AP image of incongruent varus, which also shows heterotopic ossification in the lateral gutter and syndesmosis from chronic ankle instability.

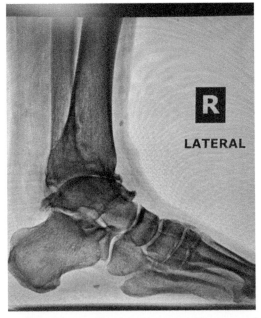

Fig. 17. Weightbearing lateral image of an incongruent ankle varus and nonreducible hindfoot deformity.

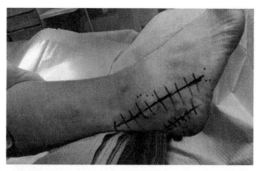

Fig. 18. Intraoperative plan for extensive lateral ankle repair including a lateralizing calcaneal osteotomy.

Varus ankle deformity is a complicated subset of ankle arthritis that has its set of risks and challenges. Focus should be on the periarticular structures, the CORA, and all ancillary procedures to get the foot plantigrade to reduce risk of failure. As with any complicated ankle deformity Case, they should be done by surgeons performing them in volume-based centers of excellence. Preoperative CT scans are recommended for most planned arthroplasty procedures which will help avoid in peri-articular cystic changes. Patient-specific instrumentation can be used to assist with deformity correction procedures and preoperative planning but is not always recommended or needed and is up to the surgical acumen and training of the treating foot and ankle physician.

VALGUS ANKLE

The Valgus ankle is the most challenging deformity when considering TAR intervention. The significance of the challenge is secondary to the intrinsic pathobiomechanics

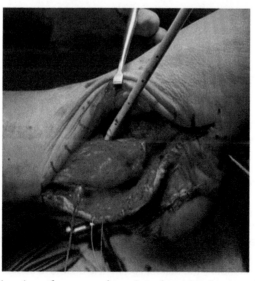

Fig. 19. Intraoperative view of a peroneal repair and revision Brostrom-Evans procedure.

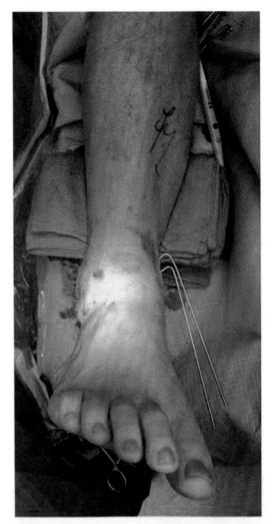

Fig. 20. Intraoperative view of an anteromedial stabilization of the ankle deformity in neutral with 2 mm Steinmann pins.

associated and kinematic manifestations persistently involved with the degenerative process. Subsequently, preoperative evaluation is of paramount importance and understanding the high-points of the deformity are essential when considering surgical intervention. Because of the insidious nature of the valgus ankle, staging the reconstructive procedure is recommended before placing the ankle replacement in most cases.

Two separate paradigms are commonly noted as driving forces in the valgus ankle. The most common is seen in the Stage IV flatfoot whereby the kinematics of the ankle are directed by severe hindfoot valgus in combination with sagittal plane collapse through the medial column. In this context, the deforming forces are translated to the ankle joint and ultimately the deltoid ligament is unable to sustain its integrity under chronic and progressive body-mass stressors.

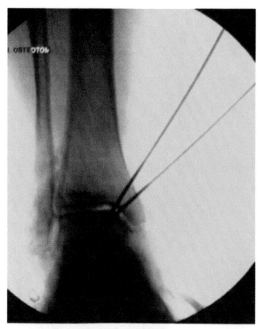

Fig. 21. Intraoperative AP view of the same patient showing the reduction in deformity.

The second paradigm is in direct consequence to a traumatic injury, most typically status postankle fracture injury, or pilon fracture whereby the deltoid ligament has been directly damaged and gone untreated; or avascular necrosis ensues to the lateral tibial plafond and collapse of the articular surface allows the talus to fall into a valgus orientation.

Delaying surgical intervention in any of these scenarios should be reserved only for those patients who are poor surgical candidates.

As it pertains to the process of staging procedures in the valgus ankle associated with Stage IV Pes Plano Valgus, the mantra of "proximal to distal and medial to lateral" is important. Any ankle equinus should be mitigated through posterior muscle group lengthening. The ankle joint then needs to be provisionally "pinned" into neutral alignment so that any reconstructive effort distally is performed around a neutral ankle mortise and preventing "overcorrection" of the flatfoot. Next osseous procedures should be performed, including but limited to hindfoot fusion or periarticular osteotomy through the subtalar joint or talonavicular joint or both. (**Fig. 24**) Next, the transverse and sagittal plane contributions of the midfoot and forefoot must be addressed, including but not limited to the navicular-cuneiform joint and or the tarsometatarsal joints. After the osseous reconstruction has commenced, then soft-tissue considerations are engaged. The deltoid ligament integrity must be restored via either allograft or autograft reconstruction or via the use of high-molecular-weight-poly-ethylene zero stretch ligament replacement. In recent years we have trended toward synthetic HMWPE implants as they are not required to incorporate into native tissue and the risk of latent attenuation is exceedingly low (**Fig. 25**). Certainly, a focus on physiologic tension with any reconstruction is paramount so as not to over-constrain or under correct at the medial ankle. Ancillary soft-tissue procedures may also be chosen, such as spring ligament repair or flexor digitorum longus tendon transfer in effort to further bolster medial ankle stability and medial column n integrity.

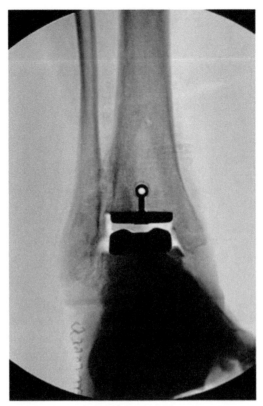

Fig. 22. Final fluoroscopic AP image of deformity reduction s/p ankle arthroplasty and peroneal tendon repair.

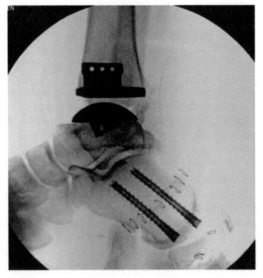

Fig. 23. Final fluoroscopic lateral image of a staged hindfoot correction and ankle arthroplasty.

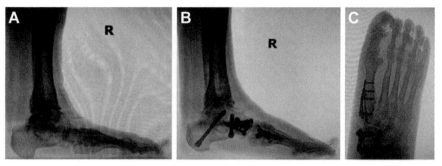

Fig. 24. (*A–C*) (foot reconstruction before TAR).

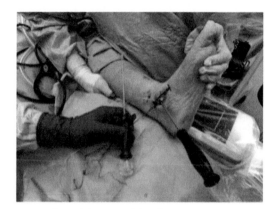

Fig. 25. Deltoid reconstruction with HMWPE implant.

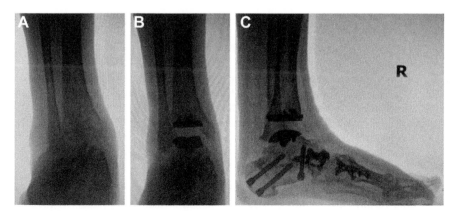

Fig. 26. (*A*) Before and (*B, C*) after staged reconstruction.

In the context of the posttraumatic ankle, all of the paradigms associated with the Stage IV flatfoot must be considered as intrinsic kinematics mirror the pathology associated. This is particularly true in scenarios whereby the patient has functioned with the valgus ankle for any significant period of time and a traumatically induced flatfoot has been driven by the valgus orientation of the ankle joint. In situations, however, whereby the tibial plafond has been worn down laterally or the avascular necrosis has directed the lateral fault, the deltoid ligament may maintain its integrity. In this scenario, the valgus deficit can be removed through the tibial cuts that are made for total ankle implantation and deformity negated through those cuts by (**Fig. 26**). Again, maintaining a mantra of "proximal to distal and medial to lateral" is of paramount importance as it pertains to procedural sequence intraoperatively.

CLINICS CARE POINTS

With an anterior approach, meticulous dissection is important without violation of the TA tendon sheath to reduce edema and soft tissue healing complications.

- Consider limited use of superficial retraction until you have performed the ankle arthrotomy and blunt dissection of the distal tibia and talus can support deep retraction.
- Tagging the extensor retinaculum on the approach for later repair may help with closure.
- Removing the tibial bone block in one piece can reduce operative time and bony fragmentation within the implantation site. Large bone pieces can get lodged posteriorly and cause posterior ankle impingement and residual pain.
- Segmenting the tibial component is sometimes necessary and one should take care to remove all fragments.
- The surgeon may want to consider having a low threshold for malleolar fixation if a stress response or occult fracture is evident intraoperatively.
- Since the so-called "learning curve" resets with each new prosthesis, ensure sound competency with any device you intend to use and train appropriately through cadaver laboratories, speaking with peers and technique reviews.
- Consider staging the ankle for a replacement in patients with multiplanar deformities (i.e., varus and valgus).
- We cannot overstate the importance of proper procedure and patient selection for this surgery.
- Understanding the need for adjunctive procedures, including GSR or tendo-Achilles lengthening, lateral or medial ligament reconstruction, or bone grafting of cystic changes, is crucial to overall success.

Expect complications and understand how to address those appropriately including revision procedures.

DISCLOSURE

J.M. Cottom Arthrex (Consultant, IP), Kinos (Consultant, IP Axiom total ankle replacement). J.G. DevriesCarbofix (Consultant), Nextremity (Consultant). C.F. Hyer Consultant/IP: Integra/Smith-Nephew, CADENCE total ankle replacement. M. Sorenson Consultant: StrykerConsultant/IP: Medline Unite. J.E. McAlister Consultant Smith + Nephew.

REFERENCES

1. Society AOFaA. Total ankle replacement (TAR). OrthopaedicsOne- The Orthopaedic Knowledge Network; 2009. p. 318–72. Available at. https://www.aofas.org/education/OrthopaedicArticles/Total-ankle-replacement.pdf.

2. Daniels TR, Younger ASE, Penner M, et al. Intermediate-term results of total ankle replacement and ankle arthrodesis: a COFAS multicenter study. J Bone Joint Surg Am 2014;96(2):135–42.
3. Schuberth JM, Patel S, Zarutsky E. Perioperative complications of the Agility total ankle replacement in 50 initial, consecutive cases. J Foot Ankle Surg 2006;45(3):139–46.
4. Schimmel JJ, Walschot LH, Louwerens JW. Comparison of the short-term results of the first and last 50 Scandanavian total ankle replacements: assessment of the learning curve in a consecutive series. Foot Ankle Int 2014;35(4):326–33.
5. Rushing CJ, McKenna BJ, Zulauf EA, et al. Intermediate-term outcomes of a third-generation, 2-component total ankle prosthesis. Foot Ankle Int 2021;42(7):935–43.
6. Mann JA, Mann RA, Horton E. STAR ankle: long-term results. Foot Ankle Int 2011;32(5):S473–84.
7. Jastifer JR, Coughlin MJ. Long-term follow-up of mobile bearing total ankle arthroplasty in the United States. Foot Ankle Int 2015;36(2):143–50.
8. Coetzee JC, Castro DM. Accurate measurement of ankle range of motion after total ankle arthroplasty. Clin Orthop Relat Res 2004;424:27–31.
9. SooHoo NF, Zingmond DS, Ko CY. Comparison of reoperation rates following ankle arthrodesis and total ankle arthroplasty. J Bone Joint Surg Am 2007;89(10):2143–9.
10. Haskell A, Mann RA. Ankle arthroplasty with preoperative coronal plane deformity: short term results. Clin Orthop Relat Res 2004;424:98–103.
11. Wood PLR, Deakin S. Total ankle replacement: the results in 200 ankles. J Bone Joint Surg Br 2003;85:334–41.
12. Saltzman CL, Salamon ML, Blanchard GM, et al. Epidemiology of ankle arthritis: report of a consecutive series of 639 patients from a tertiary orthopeadic center. Iowa Orthop J 2005;25:44–6.
13. Valderrabano V, Horisberger M, Russell I, et al. Etiology of ankle osteoarthritis. Clin Orthop Relat Res 2009;467:1800–6.
14. de Keijzer DR, Joling BSH, Sierevelt IN, et al. Influence of preoperative tibiotalar alignment in the coronal plane on the survival of total ankle replacement: a systematic review. Foot Ankle Int 2020;41(2):160–9.
15. Lee GW, Lee KB. Outcomes of total ankle arthroplasty in ankles with >20° of coronal plane deformity. J Bone Joint Surg Am 2019;101(24):2203–11.
16. Usuelli FG, Di Silvestri CA, D'Ambrosi R, et al. Total ankle replacement: is preoperative varus deformity a predictor of poor survival rate and clinical and radiological outcomes? Int Orthop 2019;43(1):243–9.

The "1-4-4-2" Model for the Diabetic Foot Team

Crystal L. Ramanujam, DPM, MSc, FACFAS*, Steven L. Stuto, DPM, Thomas Zgonis, DPM, FACFAS

KEYWORDS

- Diabetic foot team • Multidisciplinary approach • Infection • Prevention • Surgery
- Amputation

KEY POINTS

- A multidisciplinary approach should be applied in the surgical treatment of the diabetic foot to optimize each factor contributing to the overall health status of the patient.
- For the diabetic foot, it is recommended that the multidisciplinary team in the inpatient and outpatient setting should include but not limited to the following: podiatry, internal medicine, vascular surgery, cardiology, nephrology, infectious disease, endocrinology, plastic surgery, orthopedics, wound care, nursing, physical therapy, and pedorthics.
- Much like elite sports teams, skill combined with effective collaboration, clear communication, and adaptability are key components for the diabetic foot team to achieve higher rates of diabetic limb salvage.

Teamwork is an essential activity in medicine and surgery. Effective collaboration with outstanding communication and skill within an athletic team fuel victory just as these qualities facilitate successful patient outcomes within the multidisciplinary team involved in the treatment of diabetic foot complications. Dr William J. Mayo stated: "The best interest of the patient is the only interest to be considered, and in order that the sick may have the benefit of advancing knowledge, union of forces is necessary."[1] As the cause of complications in the diabetic foot is often multifactorial, treatment should include expertise from multiple branches of health care.[2] Analogous to an elite sports team, the best formation of the players on the field should be adapted based on whether the team is setting out to attack or defend. In the diabetic foot, efforts for the "defense" should be to resist ulceration, infection, amputation and/or other related complications, while the "offense" should collaborate to resolve any acute or chronic signs of infection and accomplish the ultimate goal of limb salvage. The opposing team is often intimidating and can include imposing key members

Division of Podiatric Medicine and Surgery, Department of Orthopaedics, University of Texas Health San Antonio, 7703 Floyd Curl Drive, MC 7776, San Antonio, TX 78229, USA
* Corresponding author.
E-mail address: Ramanujam@uthscsa.edu

Clin Podiatr Med Surg 39 (2022) 295–306
https://doi.org/10.1016/j.cpm.2021.11.013
0891-8422/22/© 2021 Elsevier Inc. All rights reserved.

such as gangrene, infection, peripheral vascular disease, cardiac disease, hypergly-cemia, and kidney disease. Principles of teamwork found in team sports can inform health care professionals and organizations regarding improvement in treatment stra-tegies for patients with diabetic foot complications. A large systematic review by Musuuza and colleagues[3] reported a decrease in major amputations associated with multidisciplinary teams.

THE DIABETIC FOOT TEAM

The multidisciplinary team involved in the treatment of diabetic foot complications often has several players on the field at a time like the 11 players found on a soccer team including 1 goalkeeper and 10 outfielders. The most common setup is known as the "1-4-4-2" model which has 1 goalkeeper, 4 defenders, 4 midfielders, and 2 for-wards (**Fig. 1**). While many of the players can have overlapping responsibilities and the format shape can change based on the intensity of the "game," the following descrip-tions provide the importance of each team member's role in achieving improved clin-ical and surgical outcomes when united together for a common goal.

Goalkeeper – Podiatrist/podiatric Foot and Ankle Surgeon

The *goalkeeper* always stays close to the goal to prevent the opposing team from scoring. The podiatrist/podiatric foot and ankle surgeon represents this important role and can function both in prevention and active treatment capable of providing a range of surgical options including but not limited to surgical debridement, minor amputations, foot and ankle reconstruction, plastic surgical techniques for wound closure, and prophylactic diabetic foot procedures.[4,5] They serve to quickly diagnose and determine the next "players" or consults necessary for the goal, and they often determine the direction of the entire "game" whether it goes outpatient or inpatient. Depending on the structure of the given health care system, facility and/or country, or-thopedic surgeons, diabetologists, general surgeons, vascular surgeons, or any sur-geons trained in diabetic foot surgery may serve in a similar or "back-up" role to the existing goalkeeper.

Defenders – Internists, Nursing Staff, Physical/occupational Therapy, Social Worker

Defenders do everything they can to make sure that the "ball" (ie, infection or gangrene) does not get past them. The internist provides the initial medical assess-ment and delivers baseline management of the patient's medical conditions including but not limited to hyperglycemia, hypertension, renal, and cardiac disease. The level of medical optimization required for the patient is often determined by the internist and then maintained perioperatively to help prevent complications.[6] The nursing staff pro-vides timely monitoring and delivery of important information to the entire medical team and their role as an advocate for both the patient and the physicians is vital. They assist with patient and family education and nutritional needs during the inpatient stay and in discharge planning to prepare the patient for transitioning to the outpatient setting. The physical therapy and rehabilitation medicine staff provide critical training for the patient to maintain any weight-bearing restrictions depending on the surgical procedures performed. In addition, they can provide strength training and endurance for patients to prevent deconditioning and to help determine whether further place-ment into a skilled nursing or rehabilitation center may be required. Social workers provide assistance in coordinating care for the patient's needs both inpatient and on discharge; furthermore, they can help address any psychosocial matters that might need to be addressed for the patient and their family to avoid issues that may impede

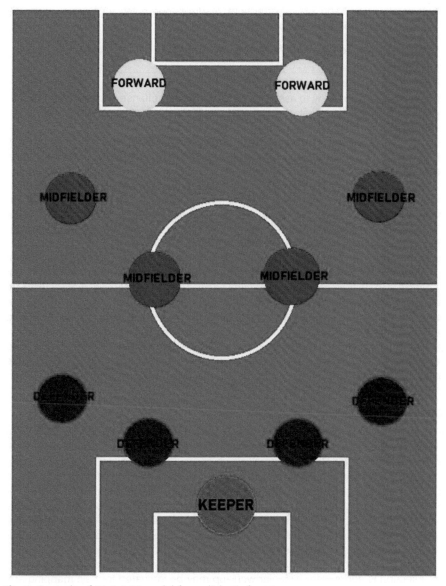

Fig. 1. Example of "1-4-4-2" model for a diabetic foot team.
Goalkeeper (1):
- Podiatrist/podiatric foot and ankle surgeon
Defenders (4):
- Internist
- Nursing staff
- Physical/Occupational therapy
- Social worker
Midfielders (4):
- Cardiologist
- Nephrologist
- Endocrinologist

postoperative care and prevent frequent readmissions given an advantage to the opposing team scoring a goal past the defenders.

Midfielders – Cardiologist, Nephrologist, Endocrinologist, Infectious Disease Specialist

Midfielders spend time playing different roles in a game to "maintain the ball" and they typically need to be ready to assist at both defense and offense. As many diabetic patients have several medical comorbidities, multiple medical issues may need to be addressed before and after surgery. For patients with cardiac valves, pacemakers, history of myocardial infarction, and cardiac interventions, the cardiologist may need to be consulted for preoperative risk stratification. Cardiac disease of new onset for a diabetic inpatient may also impact anesthesia options for diabetic foot surgery, therefore the cardiologist can be of utmost importance in determining patient and procedure selection. Renal issues in diabetic patients ranging from end-stage renal disease on hemodialysis to peritoneal dialysis to postrenal transplantation require the input of the nephrologist. Appropriate renal dosing of medications, especially antibiotics, and the management of immunosuppressive drug therapy during the perioperative period can decrease major complications. The endocrinologist provides a tight glycemic control throughout the entire "game" but also assists in the management of associated conditions such as vitamin D deficiency, osteoporosis, thyroid disease, and diabetic neuropathy. The infectious disease specialist aids with the short- and long-term parenteral intravenous or oral antibiotic therapy due to the increased finding of multiple drug-resistant organisms and involvement of both bacterial and fungal organisms in diabetic foot infections.[7] They also determine safe and cost-effective drug recommendations for the deescalation of antibiotics based on intraoperative cultures and sensitivities.

Forwards – Vascular Surgeon/Interventional Radiologist/Interventional Cardiologist, Orthopedic Surgeon/plastic Surgeon

Forwards are also known as strikers and they have the main objective of directly scoring goals. They need to be ready to attempt to score when the ball comes back their way and in diabetic foot infections, they may include vascular interventionists and plastic/orthopedic surgeons. Any suspicion of decreased perfusion or ischemic changes in the diabetic foot should be further investigated with initial noninvasive arterial testing to the lower extremities and if abnormal, a vascular interventionist should be consulted for potential angiogram with or without intervention.[3] When endovascular procedures are not a viable option, further open bypass procedures may be indicated. Continued vascular surveillance even after podiatric surgical intervention is common for these high-risk patients. In the case of plastic surgical reconstruction after the infection is addressed, vascular work-up may be indicated for vein mapping and further determination of arterial perfusion for flap design. Definitive wound closure with durable tissue that can provide function and prevent further skin breakdown and/or infection may require consultation with a plastic surgeon to provide more advanced surgical options such as microsurgical free tissue transfer.[8] The forwards are also readily available to provide treatments such as proximal leg amputations

---

- Infectious disease specialist

Forwards (2):

- Vascular surgeon/interventional radiologist/interventional cardiologist
- Orthopedic surgeon/plastic surgeon

when the team has no options or can control the "game" in urgent/emergent situations of acute sepsis due to lower extremity necrotizing infection, severe diabetic foot infections and osteomyelitis, and nonreconstructable peripheral vascular disease.

AVAILABLE TEAM MEMBERS ASSISTING THE DIABETIC FOOT TEAM

Additional members of the diabetic foot team may be "sent in" or "substituted" at any time and are available when necessary. The development of advanced imaging techniques has made musculoskeletal and nuclear imaging radiologists instrumental in differentiating conditions such as deep soft tissue and/or bone infections, with or without Charcot neuroarthropathy, and rare neoplasms.[9] Wound care specialists may assist with preventing any acute or chronic wounds of becoming infected, assist with negative pressure wound therapy, and other frequent dressing changes, reinforce the importance of non–weight-bearing status with applications of splints/casts and provide services of hyperbaric oxygen therapy when necessary. A nutritionist can help address short and/or long-term dietary issues that can affect glycemic control and to rectify deficiencies in albumin, protein, and vitamin levels.[10] Diabetes educators should be consulted during the inpatient stay to reinforce the importance of lifestyle changes that promote health and prevention of further complications. Psychologists/psychiatrists can help diabetic patients change their behaviors by controlling the blood glucose levels, adhere to their treatment regimens, address any underlying depression and psychosocial/family issues and encourage patients in a positive way for a healthier lifestyle.[11] The pedorthist/orthotist is imperative to determine accommodative shoe gear, multi-density insoles, fillers, or prostheses for partial foot or major amputations, and bracing following reconstructive surgical procedures.[12]

This multidisciplinary team concept and structure seen in the hospital inpatient setting should also be used in the outpatient setting for high-risk diabetic foot patients with the same or similar "players." Continuity of care for these patients is essential and each diabetic foot team member having knowledge regarding their own role as well as the specific roles of others on the team can make everyone more effective. Team meetings in which clear referral pathways are established and maintained as well as discussions regarding any shortcomings in processes are highly recommended for continued success.[3]

CLINICAL CASE SCENARIOS WITH A DIABETIC FOOT TEAM "STARTING LINE-UP"
Prophylactic, Elective, and Reconstructive Surgery

The "starting line-up" and/or "model/format" for the diabetic foot team in cases of prophylactic, elective, and reconstructive diabetic foot surgery might have to change according to the patient's characteristics and associated medical conditions, lower extremity deformity, surgical procedure, rehabilitation, and available medical/surgical specialties with an interest in the management of the diabetic foot (**Fig. 2**).

For example, in a patient with a chronic and unstable Charcot neuroarthropathy of the foot or ankle that is being preoperatively prepared for surgical reconstruction, the podiatric foot, and ankle surgeon (*goalkeeper*) promptly initiates a full workup and consults with the *defenders* that have a new role in this "game" and may include the internist/primary care physician, cardiologist, endocrinologist and vascular surgeon (**Fig. 3**). Note that in this particular clinical case scenario that the diabetic foot team "players" may initially be needed in different positions for the safety of the patient and to achieve the goal of a successful recovery. The *midfielders* may consist of diabetic foot team "players" from nephrology, infectious disease, physical therapy, and nursing staff during the patient's hospital stay. The *forwards* may include the social

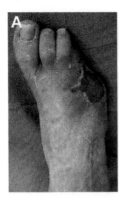
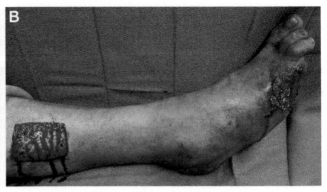

Fig. 2. Preoperative photograph (*A*) of a diabetic patient who was scheduled for a recon-structive surgical procedure of an autogenous split-thickness skin graft harvested from the right leg to the right foot (*B*). The diabetic foot team on this model will maintain the podiatric foot and ankle surgeon as the *goalkeeper* who promptly initiates a full workup and consults with their *teammates* before the definitive surgery.

worker and pedorthist/orthotist that will help with the patient's transition of care. The inpatient social worker (*forward*) coordinates discharge needs for smooth transfer to the rehabilitation facility and helps obtain assistive devices for postoperative care. The podiatric foot and ankle surgeon (*goalkeeper*) continue care in the outpatient setting and continues to assist in reaching the final goal of ambulation long-term in custom diabetic shoe gear with bracing designed by a pedorthist/orthotist (*forward*).

Available team members to be sent in or substituted at any time for this diabetic foot team may include but are not limited to members from musculoskeletal/nuclear imaging radiology, wound care specialists, nutritionists, or diabetes educators.

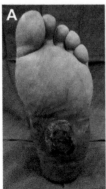
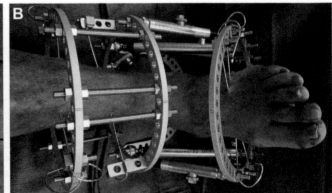

Fig. 3. Preoperative photograph (*A*) of a diabetic patient who was scheduled for a recon-structive surgical procedure of a right foot Charcot neuroarthropathy (*B*). The diabetic foot team on this model will still maintain the podiatric foot and ankle surgeon as the *goalkeeper* who promptly initiates a full workup and consults with their *teammates* before the definitive surgery. Due to the complexity of the case and patient's underlying medical conditions, the *starting line-up* might have to be changed and adjusted according to the pre-operative testing and *teammates* recommendations.

Urgent/emergent Diabetic Foot Surgery

The "starting line-up" and/or "model/format" for the diabetic foot team in cases of urgent/emergent diabetic foot surgery is based on the severity of the diabetic foot infection and associated medical comorbidities. The podiatrist/podiatric foot and ankle surgeon is the *goalkeeper* and sees the entire "game" by initiating the appropriate consultations and hospital admission. The *defenders* of the diabetic foot team during the hospitalization may include the internist, infectious disease specialist, physical therapist, and social worker, while the *midfielders* may consist of team members from cardiology, nephrology, musculoskeletal radiology, and nutrition and *forwards* may include the vascular interventionist and pedorthist/orthotist (**Figs. 4 and 5**).

For example, a diabetic patient who is presenting to the emergency room with clinical, radiographic and systemic signs of infection, osteomyelitis and sepsis is consulted initially by the podiatrist/podiatric foot and ankle surgeon (*goalkeeper*) who is directing the hospital admission, surgical procedure(s) and appropriate consultations. The hospitalist (*defender*) manages the patient's medical conditions, provides medical optimization, and maintains appropriate glycemic control. Physical therapy (*defender*)

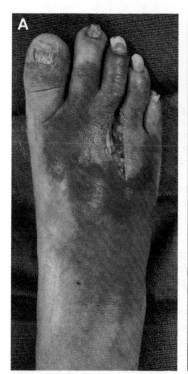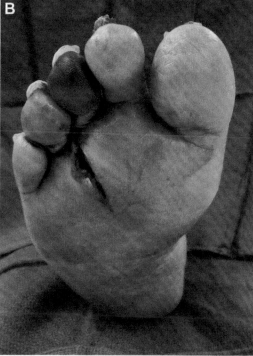

Fig. 4. Postoperative photographs (*A, B*) of a diabetic patient who underwent an incision and drainage for a diabetic foot infection during the initial hospitalization that developed ischemic changes to the third toe. The diabetic foot team on this model will maintain the podiatric foot and ankle surgeon as the *goalkeeper* who promptly initiates a full workup and consults with their *teammates* during the hospital stay and before the multiple staged surgical procedures. Due to the complexity/urgency of the case and patient's underlying medical conditions, the *starting line-up* is changed and adjusted according to the patient's needs and *teammates'* recommendations.

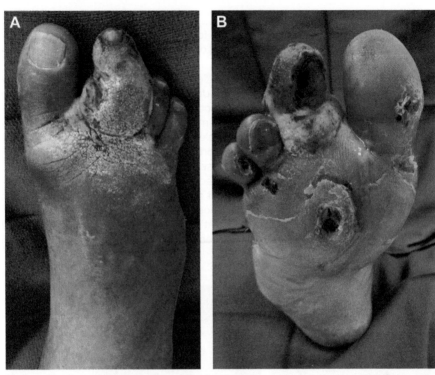

Fig. 5. Preoperative photographs (*A, B*) of a diabetic patient who presented to the emergency room with a severe diabetic foot infection, osteomyelitis, and sepsis. The diabetic foot team on this model will maintain the podiatric foot and ankle surgeon as the *goalkeeper* who promptly initiates a full workup and consults with their *teammates* during the hospital stay and before the multiple staged surgical procedures to avoid a major lower extremity amputation. Due to the urgency/emergency of the case and patient's underlying medical conditions, the *starting line-up* is changed and adapted in a quick and efficient way for a medical/surgical decision and according to the patient's needs and *teammates* recommendations.

is consulted for weight-bearing restrictions with assistive devices, while the infectious disease specialist (*defender*) and social worker (*defender*) will coordinate the duration and delivery of antibiotic therapy and work on hospital discharge planning.

Medical imaging by musculoskeletal radiology (*midfielder*) includes plain radiographs, computed tomography of the lower extremity to assess for gas, or magnetic resonance imaging to evaluate for residual soft tissue and bone infection. The rest of the team (*midfielders*) may include a cardiologist based on the patient's cardiac disease, type of anesthesia and surgical procedure, nephrologist based on the patient's kidney disease and/or hemodialysis and nutritionist based on the patient's overall medical status and uncontrolled blood sugars. Clinical findings of ischemia, gangrene, and minimal intraoperative bleeding along with confirmed moderate-to-severe arterial occlusive disease based on noninvasive arterial testing warrants a vascular surgery consultation (*forward*) and further endovascular versus open bypass procedures. On successful recovery and ambulation, diabetic extra depth shoes with custom multidensity insoles and filler(s) for any type of amputation by a pedorthist/orthotist (*forward*) is managed for a long-term follow-up.

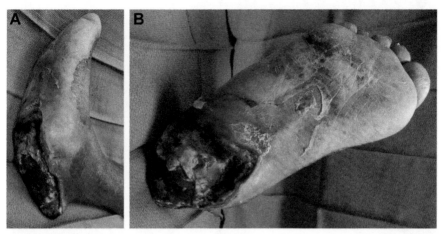

Fig. 6. Preoperative photographs (*A*, *B*) of a diabetic patient who initially presented to the emergency room with a severe diabetic foot infection, osteomyelitis, gas gangrene and sepsis that underwent multiple excisional debridements. The diabetic foot team on this model will have to make some significant changes on the *starting line-up* and assign a new *goalkeeper* who will direct the hospital admission, urgent/emergent surgical proced-ure(s) including but not limited to lower extremity amputation and appropriate consultations.

Limb/life-Threatening Diabetic Foot Surgery

The "starting line-up" for the diabetic foot team in cases of limb/life-threatening dia-betic foot surgery has to be organized in an expedited time whereby the podiatrist/ podiatric foot and ankle surgeon (*goalkeeper*) who is initially consulted might have to be "substituted" by his teammate orthopedic, vascular, general, or plastic surgeon depending on the specialty availability, facilities, and/or geographic region/country. The newly assigned *goalkeeper* will then direct the hospital admission, surgical pro-cedure(s)) including but not limited to lower extremity amputation and appropriate consultations (**Figs. 6 and 7**).

For example, a patient who presents to the emergency department with severe sepsis, leukocytosis, gas gangrene, necrotizing infection, and pain extending from the foot into the leg will have a new *goalkeeper* as discussed previously with a different diabetic foot team format. The *defenders* may include the hospitalist, infectious dis-ease specialist, physical therapist, and social worker, while the *midfielders* may include the cardiologist, nephrologist, psychologist/psychiatrist, and nutritionist. The *forwards* may include the pedorthist/orthotist for the planning of the prosthesis and podiatrist/podiatric foot and ankle surgeon who manages the contralateral limb pre-venting any contralateral lower extremity complications.

REFEREE AND LINESMAN

The main duty of a *referee* who is the anesthesiologist is to make sure the "game" is not delayed or postponed and enforce patient safety. The *referee* monitors the pa-tient's safety and can stop or terminate the "game" due to multiple risk factors and are also in charge of keeping time during the "game". For the diabetic foot team that is ready to proceed with the proposed surgical procedure, the anesthesiologist is the referee and the certified registered nurse anesthetists (CRNAs) serve as linesman or assistant referees. The anesthesiologist has the final say in whether the

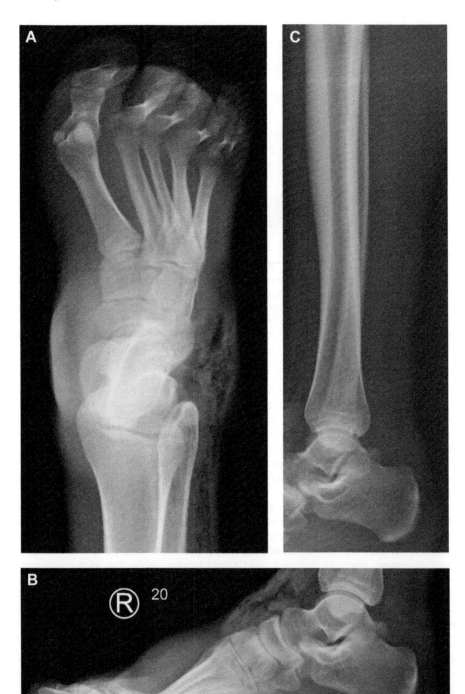

surgery can proceed or not, effectively in control of the entire "game". A cardiac anesthesiologist may be recommended to "referee" for high-risk cardiac patients and this is determined early in the preoperative process so that their availability can be coordinated with the time of surgery.

COACH/TEACHER

The coach is responsible for guiding each team member individually and together as a team. They determine whether the team focuses on either defensive or offensive play depending on the given situation in a game. The coach/teacher for the multidisciplinary diabetic foot team is the "game" itself and all of its clinical manifestations. Diabetes mellitus (*coach/teacher*) will test the team members to identify their strengths and weaknesses, become proactive with better communication skills, reflect on their performance, and in turn, all the team members learn from the disease to define each of their specific roles.

KEY QUALITIES FOR ESTABLISHING AN ELITE DIABETIC FOOT TEAM

A patient-centered approach allows the diabetic foot team to work in an environment that is constantly based on the characteristics of the specific patient being treated. This allows each team member to analyze the "game" and use their unique expertise to make decisions that are beneficial to the goal of preventing or saving a diabetic lower extremity from being amputated. The team members are left to exercise critical thinking and can be creative with their own solutions.

All members of the team should be chosen for their shared vision in caring for diabetic patient. They should be proactive with quick decision-making and ready to adapt their treatment path to any changes in the treatment plan. Shared "goals" and vision for the entire team in addition to a strong sense of responsibility to the patient and patient's family are imperative for effective collaboration and group success. The diabetic foot team should take time for inpatient and outpatient meetings which allows for self-reflection and continuous learning based on patient outcomes. Discussion of any specific highlights or pitfalls for each patient can show each team member how to enhance or duplicate the positive moves and improve on the negative ones.

In the inpatient setting, collaboration with teaching rounds, lectures/conferences, and leadership within the facility/institution will further enhance the teamwork model to be successful for the patient's goal of a healthy recovery. In the outpatient setting, combined clinics in which several members of the multidisciplinary team are present simultaneously to provide treatment and coordinate plans are another chance to actively put into effect those qualities learned through times of reflection and also emphasize the patient-centered approach. Long-term goals of establishing centers of excellence for patients with diabetic foot complications are the ultimate solution

---

Fig. 7. Preoperative radiographs (*A–C*) of a diabetic patient who initially presented to the emergency room with a severe diabetic foot infection, gas gangrene of the lower extremity, and sepsis that underwent an urgent/emergent below-the-knee amputation. The diabetic foot team on this model was changed in an expedited time and assigned a new *goalkeeper* who directed the hospital admission, urgent/emergent surgical procedure, and appropriate consultations.

for all health care members to collaborate efficiently in an organized and safe environment with a patient-centered approach.

SUMMARY

While the concept of a "team" in medicine is not new, the specific structure of the multidisciplinary team for diabetic foot infections and the ability for the entire team to adapt together in fluid situations should be emphasized for improved clinical outcomes in limb salvage. As seen in elite team sports, sheer talent and skill must be accompanied by effective communication, shared values, and commitment to collaboration as the foundation for a successful multidisciplinary team in treating diabetic foot infections.

REFERENCES

1. Mayo foundation for medical education and research 1910: the best interest of the patient. Available at; http://history.mayoclinic.org/toolkit/quotations/the-doctors-mayo.php.
2. Frykberg RG. The team approach in diabetic foot management. Adv Wound Care 1998;11(2):71–7.
3. Musuuza J, Sutherland BL, Kurter S, et al. A systematic review of multidisciplinary teams to reduce major amputations for patients with diabetic foot ulcers. J Vasc Surg 2020;71(4):1433–46.e3.
4. Frykberg RG, Zgonis T, Armstrong DG, et al, American College of Foot and Ankle Surgeons. Diabetic foot disorders. A clinical practice guideline (2006 revision). J Foot Ankle Surg 2006;45(5 Suppl):S1–66.
5. Frykberg RG, Wittmayer B, Zgonis T. Surgical management of diabetic foot infections and osteomyelitis. Clin Podiatr Med Surg 2007;24(3):469–82, viii–ix.
6. Ayada G, Edel Y, Burg A, et al. Multidisciplinary team led by internists improves diabetic foot ulceration outcomes a before-after retrospective study. Eur J Intern Med 2021;94:64–8. https://doi.org/10.1016/j.ejim.2021.07.007.
7. Chastain CA, Klopfenstein N, Serezani CH, et al. A clinical review of diabetic foot infections. Clin Podiatr Med Surg 2019;36(3):381–95.
8. Lee ZH, Daar DA, Stranix JT, et al. Free-flap reconstruction for diabetic lower extremity limb salvage. J Surg Res 2020;248:165–70.
9. Short DJ, Zgonis T. Medical imaging in differentiating the diabetic Charcot foot from osteomyelitis. Clin Podiatr Med Surg 2017;34(1):9–14.
10. Brookes JDL, Jaya JS, Tran H, et al. Broad-ranging nutritional deficiencies predict amputation in diabetic foot ulcers. Int J Low Extrem Wounds 2020;19(1):27–33.
11. Roukis TS, Stapleton JJ, Zgonis T. Addressing psychosocial aspects of care for patients with diabetes undergoing limb salvage surgery. Clin Podiatr Med Surg 2007;24(3):601–10, xi.
12. Koller A. Internal pedal amputations. Clin Podiatr Med Surg 2008;25(4):641–53, ix.

Surgical Treatment of Diabetic Foot and Ankle Osteomyelitis

Kimia Sohrabi, DPM[a],*, Ronald Belczyk, DPM[b]

KEYWORDS

- Osteomyelitis • Diagnosis • Treatment • Diabetic foot • Academic center

KEY POINTS

- Osteomyelitis (OM) is a common disease that presents in the foot and ankle with clinical microbiological varieties.
- Multispecialty management of osteomyelitis is the mainstay method of treatment in an academic setting.
- Early diagnosis is needed to initiate treatment.

Osteomyelitis is a common disease that presents in the foot and ankle with clinical and microbiological varieties. Although the goal is to cure patients with osteomyelitis, it can be challenging for numerous reasons. Early detection is important to prevent chronic infections and complications, and early identification can also be difficult.

The patient's age, mechanism of injury or contamination, and medications may affect the clinical and diagnostic features of the disease process. Management of osteomyelitis in the foot and ankle can be challenging from both medical and surgical perspectives due to possible clinical presentations with ulceration, soft tissue infection, gangrene, polymicrobial infections, compromised circulation, instability of joints, fracture or dislocation, and noncompliance of patients. In addition, the ability to deliver antibiotics to the distal skeleton in vascular-compromised patients, need for long-term antibiotics, and side effects with long-term medications in compromised hosts with renal comorbidities may also challenge the treatment of osteomyelitis. Bacteria exhibit multiple factors that contribute to the severity and chronicity of osteomyelitis. Bacterial proteins known as adhesins attach bacteria to bone, and the formation of glycocalyx-rich biofilm makes the bacteria less susceptible to antibiotics; both features can contribute to severity and chronicity of infection.

Multispecialty management of osteomyelitis is the mainstay method of treatment in an academic setting. Collaborative involvement between infectious disease, podiatry,

[a] Foot and Ankle Centers of North Houston, 17215 Red Oak Drive #102, Houston, TX 77090, USA; [b] Center for Foot Surgery, Oxnard, 903 West 7th Street, Oxnard, CA 93030, USA
* Corresponding author.
E-mail address: Dr.kimiasohrabi@gmail.com

Clin Podiatr Med Surg 39 (2022) 307–319
https://doi.org/10.1016/j.cpm.2021.11.003
0891-8422/22/© 2021 Elsevier Inc. All rights reserved.

pathology, and any other medical and surgical teams needed for consultation can prove a more effective and definitive treatment of osteomyelitis, which allows for a better knowledge of antibiotic treatment duration and role of oral antibiotics in managing osteomyelitis.[1] Infections often complicated by bacterial biofilms will reduce the efficacy of antibiotics. Long-term use of antibiotics may have negative side effects such as nephrotoxicity, thus, patients would also benefit from a nephrology consultation when necessary. Peripheral arterial disease can reduce the effectiveness of systemic antimicrobial therapy due to poor local tissue perfusion. Unfortunately, this may result in antibiotic levels not reaching the minimal inhibitory contribution of the pathogens at the site of infection. Peripheral angiography and intervention with angioplasty or lower extremity bypass may be needed in the vascular-compromised patients. Once patients are transitioned from the acute setting to either skilled nursing or home, the community nursing staff can assist with home evaluation, delivery of antibiotics, and reporting of further complications.[2] In cases with ulcer resolution, underlying osteomyelitis is considered to be in remission.

CLINICAL PRESENTATION

Osteomyelitis in the foot and ankle can be acute or chronic and can involve cortical and/or intramedullary bone.[3] Osteomyelitis can present as contiguous, hematogenous, or disseminated forms[4,5] (**Fig. 1**).

The clinical presentation varies based on the type of infection, chronicity, anatomic location, and comorbidities of the host. Surgical wound dehiscence, edema, and exposed hardware create portals for infection, which can lead to delayed wound

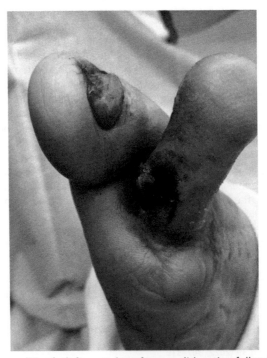

Fig. 1. Acute osteomyelitis of a left second toe fracture dislocation following minor injury in a patient with type 1 diabetes mellitus with peripheral neuropathy.

healing, granulation, and often osteomyelitis. Patients with osteomyelitis in the acute setting may present with fever, chills, pain, edema, inflammation, and purulent drainage from an open wound. Severe infection may present with gas within the soft tissues and be rapidly spreading along fascial planes.

Osteomyelitis in the chronic setting can occur in patients who are not systemically ill and often have symptoms for weeks or months. Following surgery with implantation of orthopedic hardware, the clinical findings for osteomyelitis can be subtle such as mild edema, local pain, and erythema. If the underlying bone cannot be probed, it does not exclude the diagnosis of osteomyelitis. Delayed radiographic union is not normal for fracture healing or arthrodesis. On other case scenarios, surgical wound dehiscence with chronically exposed hardware or bone is highly suspicious for osteomyelitis and warrants further investigation.

DIAGNOSTIC WORKUP

Early diagnosis is needed to initiate treatment. Several imaging modalities are useful in the evaluation of osteomyelitis including radiographs, bone scintigraphy, computed tomography (CT), and MRI. Radiographs are easily obtainable, inexpensive, and safe. Early radiographic changes include soft tissue changes such as edema or ulceration. Comparison radiographs of the contralateral extremity can be helpful. However, periosteal reaction and bone necrosis may not be seen initially, and negative radiographic findings do not exclude the diagnosis of osteomyelitis in the acute setting. Osseous changes may not be evident for 10 to 14 days or until 35% to 50% of the bone is destroyed.[6,7]

With contiguous osteomyelitis, the infection first involves the tissue, periosteum, cortex, and then the medullary bone. With hematogenous spread osteomyelitis, the medullary bone is first affected. With chronic osteomyelitis, a sclerotic layer of bone can form around a sequestrum. Necrotic islands of bone, Brodie abscess, and granulation can be seen near the sequestrum. Bacterial infections have similar radiographic findings, whereas mycobacterial and fungal infections can demonstrate unique findings. Serial radiographic imaging can be obtained after surgery or fracture to monitor the progress of bone healing. With comminuted fracture patterns, the bone fragments may have poor vascularity and may resemble sequestra. Prolonged cast immobilization may demonstrate osteoporotic changes. Although some situations may require additional imaging modalities, plain radiographs have a sensitivity of 43% to 75% and specificity of 75% to 83%.[8,9] When positive radiographic findings are demonstrated, then biopsy, culture, and/or surgical intervention can be recommended modalities for treatment.

When radiographs are inconclusive and there is a high index of suspicion for osteomyelitis, then bone scintigraphy with a radioisotope can be performed, typically with technetium-99m methylene diphosphate, gallium-67, indium-111, or technetium 99m-hexamethylpropyleneamine oxime-labeled leukocytes. Osteomyelitis demonstrates increased tracer accumulation in all 3 phases. The technetium-99 m hexamethylpropyleneamine oxime-labeled leukocytes have been used to detect early infection. Three-phase bone scan has a sensitivity of 73% to 100% and specificity of 73% to 79%.[8,9] Because lymphocytes are not labeled, there is a reduced sensitivity in chronic infections and spatial resolution may not provide anatomic details needed for surgical planning.

When greater anatomic detail is needed, a CT or MRI can be performed.

CT scans can be used to detect early bone erosions, sequestrum, foreign bodies, and emphysema. CT has a sensitivity of 65% to 75% and specificity of 65% to

75%.[8,9] A technetium 99m-hexamethylpropyleneamine oxime white blood cell single-photon emission CT/CT could be useful in assessing diabetic foot osteomyelitis in remission. This method can distinguish between residual infections and postinflammatory uptake.[10]

MRI is helpful with enhanced image quality and characterization of bone infections. Studies can be performed with or without contrast. Osteomyelitis can be seen as low signal intensity in marrow on T1-weighted sequences and seen as high signal intensity in marrow on T2-weighted sequences. In T2-weighted sequences the fat signal is suppressed and is more helpful in evaluating cortical bone. MRI has a sensitivity of 80% to 90% and specificity of 80% to 90%.[8,9] MRI can be limited when a patient's body habitus and movement during the study results in unclear images. Also, internal fixation can result in local image distortion and can be more challenging to interpret in cases with previous surgery and chronic infection without identifiable fluid collections or sinus tracts.

Blood tests are typically performed in the evaluation and management of bone infection. Many compromised hosts fail to have an elevated white blood cell count. Blood cultures are only positive in about 50% of patients.[11,12] Erythrocyte sedimentation rate (ESR) and C-reactive protein (CRP) are the routinely ordered inflammatory biomarkers for evaluating foot infection. Both lack the specificity without imaging and culture results. Some autoimmune disorders could affect the ESR and CRP levels; however, both tests can be obtained to monitor response to antibiotics and surgery. An ESR of 60 mm/h and CRP level of 7.9 mg/dL were determined to be the optimal cutoff points for predicting osteomyelitis.[13] If the ESR is less than 30 mm/h, the likelihood of osteomyelitis is low. However, if the ESR is greater than60 mm/h and CRP is greater than 7.9 mg/dL, the likelihood of osteomyelitis is high and treatment of suspected osteomyelitis should be considered.[13] ESR is better for ruling out osteomyelitis initially, whereas CRP helps distinguish osteomyelitis from soft tissue infection in patients with high ESR values.[13]

Procalcitonin (PCT) may serve as a useful marker for diagnosing diabetic foot osteomyelitis. A pilot study with PCT in distinguishing between diabetic foot osteomyelitis and cellulitis demonstrated a 79% sensitivity and 70% specificity.[14] PCT levels were 0.13 ± 0.02 ng/mL in patients with diabetic osteomyelitis and 0.04 ± 0.02 ng/mL in patients without osteomyelitis. The best cutoff value for PCT was 0.085 ng/mL.[15] PCT, ESR, and CRP values are higher in patients with osteomyelitis ($P < .001$).[15] PCT is a useful diagnostic test for diabetic foot osteomyelitis and can be used to differentiate it from cellulitis.[14]

MANAGEMENT

Management of osteomyelitis depends on the pathogen identification and host characteristics. Percutaneous or open biopsy can be performed to identify the infecting organisms. If the infection is severe and the lower extremity is not salvageable, then complete resection of the infected bones or more proximal-level amputation is considered.

In the Western countries, gram-positive bacteria are the most commonly encountered pathogens. Pathogen identification and sensitivity is important to use proper antibiotics.[16] *Staphylococcus aureus* is seen in 81% to 92% of cases from hematogenous spread osteomyelitis.[17] Beta-hemolytic streptococcal infections have been reported in children.[18] *Escherichia coli, Pseudomonas aeruginosa, Klebsiella, and Aerobacter* species are often encountered in patients with comorbidities such as alcoholism, sickle cell, or diabetes.[7,17,19] Fungal osteomyelitis is uncommon in the foot and ankle but can be considered in patients with diabetes, those on chronic steroids, and in immunocompromised patients.

Targeted antibiotic therapy for diabetic foot osteomyelitis should be based on antimicrobial susceptibility testing in bone and soft tissue cultures.[20] Histopathological analysis provides more accurate diagnosis of diabetic foot osteomyelitis than microbiological examination, especially for patients with chronic diabetic foot osteomyelitis. Patients could also be underdiagnosed because of false-negative results provided by bone cultures.[21]

Genetic testing may be more sensitive and specific than traditional methods and provide results faster than other techniques such as cultures. For instance, nucleic acid amplification, like with polymerase chain reaction, makes numerous copies of any genetic material from the microbes present in a sample so that it can be more easily detected. Genetic testing can be used to determine the type of microbe present. Some genetic tests identify specific genes that enable a microbe to grow in the presence of an antimicrobial drug or identify a genotype of bacteria that will respond to specific treatment. For instance, E coli from diabetic foot infections and osteomyelitis was assessed for clonal diversity, resistance profile, virulence potential, and genome adaptation. A shared mutation was observed on both strains; however, E coli from osteomyelitis were genetically diverse with varying pathogenicity traits; their adaptation in the bone structure could require genome reduction and modification.[22]

The medical management of osteomyelitis requires early diagnosis, selecting appropriate antibiotics, and determining which cases require surgery. Empirical antibiotic therapy not guided by culture results is likely to be ineffective. There may be some situations in which it is not safe to remove the implanted internal fixation, prosthesis, or necrotic bone, so it may be necessary to treat the patient with long-term antibiotics for suppression of infection. However, there are numerous potential side effects and concerns for antibiotic resistance with suppressive antibiotics including nephrotoxicity and ototoxicity. Generally, a combined medical and surgical approach is the preferred method for treatment of osteomyelitis.

A high clinical or radiographic suspicion of osteomyelitis may indicate the need for bone biopsy to identify the involved organisms and antibiotic sensitivity. A percutaneous or open biopsy of bone is performed to obtain specimens for microbiology and histopathology analyses to determine the pathogens or evaluate for clean surgical margins. The primary goal with surgical debridement is to remove the necrotic bone because poorly vascularized bone most likely will not heal. Some case considerations for management of osteomyelitis that need to be discussed include diabetic osteomyelitis, osteomyelitis in the presence of soft tissue infection, implanted hardware, and infection of the calcaneus.

SURGICAL APPROACHES TO OSTEOMYELITIS

Recent studies have shown rates of remission of diabetic osteomyelitis and reulceration after treatment. A systematic review of the literature shows that treatment of diabetic osteomyelitis requires selection of appropriate modality based on the indication and characteristics of the patient.[23] Lower rates of remission in patients with diabetic foot osteomyelitis undergoing surgical treatment have been found.[23] In respect to reulceration, Tardaguila-Garcia and colleagues[24] looked at osteomyelitis cases of the forefoot. In a 1-year follow-up, the onset of complications after surgical or medical treatment of osteomyelitis in the forefoot did not show a significant difference between the 2 cohorts. The most common complication in both groups was reulceration. Surgical and medical approaches to the management of predominantly forefoot osteomyelitis produced similar results in a long-term follow-up.[24]

Because patients with peripheral neuropathy remain ambulatory, foot and ankle deformities of the forefoot remain a contributing factor. Abnormal gait patterns cannot be negated with over-the-counter footwear, and in some case, customized prosthesis. Hammertoes contribute to pressure at dorsal interphalangeal joints and distal aspect of the toes. Conservative surgery is an alternative to amputation and strives to preserve functionality of the foot. Many patients adamantly refuse amputation. Conservative surgery, also known as foot-sparing surgery, means resecting only the infected and necrotic bone without amputating. This surgery also has advantages by reducing the duration of antibiotics and selecting evidence-based antibiotic regimens, often of a limited pathogen spectrum.[25] Internal pedal amputation as salvage procedure in diabetic and ischemic foot infections is thought to be helpful with removing the infected bone while preserving the underlying anatomy. Conservative surgery was not associated with a lower rate of recurrence than those who underwent amputations.[26]

The goal of an amputation is to eradicate infection while leaving a functional foot for ambulation; this often involves disarticulating at the joint proximal to the affected bone. This concept becomes complicated when metatarsals are involved, because they contribute to most of the foot's length. The most affected part of the metatarsals is often resected, with the hopes of leaving clean proximal bone margins, which is often confirmed through proximal margin bone biopsies.

Patients with moderate osteomyelitis have a high rate of recurrence after initial treatment and require longer time to heal when compared with moderate soft tissue infections. No differences were seen between severe infections with or without osteomyelitis in regard to limb loss rate, length of hospital stays, duration of antibiotic treatment, recurrence of infection, and time to healing[26] (Fig. 2).

Osteomyelitis is difficult to eradicate in the presence of implanted hardware.

There are several risk factors that contribute to deep infection rates of the foot and ankle after open reduction and internal fixation (ORIF), which includes alcoholism, age, diabetes, and high-energy injuries. Some argue that overall complications and union rates are similar between ORIF and closed reduction using external fixation. However, the presence of extensive soft tissue compromise can be a good indication for the use of external fixation to reduce high-energy open fracture complications.[4,5]

When encountering postoperative ankle infection, eradicating the infection is the primary objective, and then if possible, restoring foot and ankle function. Once infected hardware is extracted and osteolytic bone is resected, an extensive osseous deficit is often created. In conjunction with intravenous antibiotics, impregnated antibiotic cements as beads or block spacers are used to maintain soft tissue tension and joint stability. Once the infection is eradicated and the implanted antibiotic drug delivery system is removed, the involved joints can be prepared for arthrodesis and stabilization using internal or external fixation. When extensive bone loss is present in the ankle joint, external fixation technique is the ideal method to correct limb length discrepancy by means of proximal lengthening while simultaneously fusing the distal joints by means of compression[3] (Fig. 3).

The calcaneus is a delicate anatomic structure when injury occurs and can have profound effect on long-term function. Many times, osteomyelitis is preceded by calcaneal gait patterns from weak plantarflexion, previous tendo-Achilles lengthening or ruptures, and calcaneal fractures, which often lead to increased pressure at the plantar hindfoot. Chronic ulcerations of the heel can lead to contiguous spread of bacteria to the cortex of the calcaneus. Progression of infection and weight-bearing can lead to pathologic fractures of the calcaneus and septic arthritis of the subtalar joint. The biomechanically unsound foot due to instability of joints, fracture and/or dislocation, malunion, or Charcot neuroarthropathy can pose challenges to both medical and

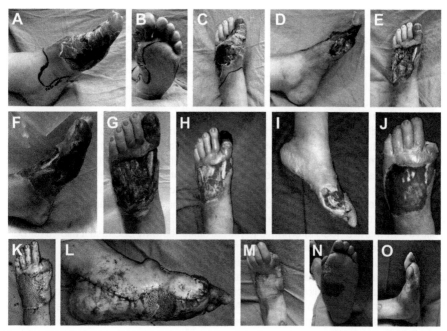

Fig. 2. Initial puncture wound presentation involving acute osteomyelitis of the hallux with extensive soft tissue infection (*A–C*). Puncture wound following incision and drainage and debridement of soft tissue infection (*D, E*). Demarcation of infection (*F–H*) required partial amputation of hallux (*I, J*). Wound closure of the open amputation site with a reverse flow medial plantar artery flap and autogenous split-thickness skin grafting (*K, L*). Final healed outcome (*M–O*).

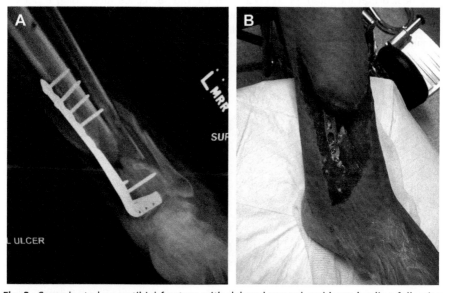

Fig. 3. Comminuted open tibial fracture with delayed wound and bone healing following open reduction and internal fixation (*A, B*). Despite extensive tissue and bone defects patient was refusing major limb amputation.

surgical treatments (**Fig. 4**). For a more favorable surgical outcome, it is often preferable to preoperatively optimize the patient's nutritional status, glycemic control, and anemia before resection of any portion of the calcaneus. The amount of resection is often determined by the extent of the osteomyelitis in the bone, wound size, and the location within the calcaneus.[27,28] There are 3 favored surgical techniques for treatment of calcaneal osteomyelitis: bone preservation, bone destruction/partial calcanectomy, and vertical contour calcanectomy.[27,29]

The bone preservation method includes debridement of the necrotic and nonviable soft tissue, drilling 6 to 9 holes in the calcaneus and inserting gentamicin sulfate pegs. The bone destruction method allows for radical debridement of all infected osteomyelitic bone. Elmarsafi and colleagues[27] concluded that although bone preservation method is a viable alternative, a more proximal amputation or partial calcanectomy allows for better source control, more patient satisfaction, and comparable walking ability. Vertical contouring involves detaching the Achilles tendon and plantar fascia, performing 3 cardinal osteotomies with contouring, and closure. The investigators believe that this is a good alternative to partial calcanectomy because it allows for better primary closure and bone coverage.[27]

Minimal bone resection from the plantar calcaneus results in a more functional biomechanical outcome because the calcaneus maintains the integrity of its weight-bearing surface, which allows for a functional Achilles tendon and less weakening of the posterior muscle group[30,31] (**Fig. 5**). At the same time, failure to eradicate the infection by means of minimal resection can lead to a more proximal infection and possible limb loss.[32] A study by Oliver and colleagues,[32] showed that the below-the-knee amputation rate had no statistical significance between patients who had less than 50% of the calcaneus resected and those who had greater than 50% of the calcaneus resected.

Chronic osteomyelitis, although rare, can lead to calcaneal fractures, which results in more proximal amputations like below-the-knee amputation. Some investigators hypothesize that the interruption created in the biomechanics after doing a plantar instead of vertical calcaneal excision and sparing the Achilles attachment can lead to the posterior muscle group overwhelming the dorsal calcaneal cortex to cause calcaneal fractures.[32,33]

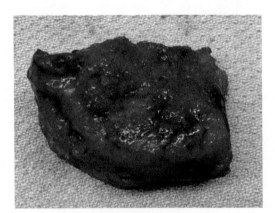

Fig. 4. Intraoperative photograph showing the resection of a calcaneal bone. Clinical features of the excised bone include discoloration, granuloma, moth-eaten cortical bone erosion, and purulence from bone.

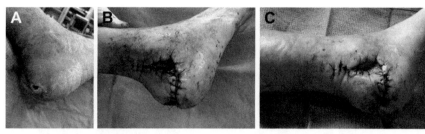

Fig. 5. Chronic calcaneus osteomyelitis (*A*) with local involvement treated with bone resection and short version of a pedicled lateral calcaneal artery flap (*B, C*).

In these circumstances, internal fixation should not be used and due to the integrity of the bone, reduction with external fixation is rendered very difficult. If it is feasible, fracture fragments can be excised, but this can cause further instability, especially if the Achilles tendon is involved. Therefore, fracture excision can have less than a favorable surgical outcome with a nonfunctional foot or a calcaneal gait. Not reducing the fracture can lead to further tissue damage and less-than-desirable outcomes.[34] It is also estimated that 25% of all calcaneal fractures lead to soft tissue complications.[35] Depending on the location of the soft tissue deficit, the exposed calcaneus can be closed by other methods such as adjacent tissue transfer, perforator flaps, fasciocutaneous flaps, musculofasciocutaneous flaps, free flaps, or negative pressure therapy with subsequent skin grafting[36,37] (**Fig. 6**).

Local delivery of antibiotics has been used to minimize systemic toxicity and eliminate concerns about antibiotic penetration while achieving high local doses of antibiotics. A retrospective study reviewing surgical cases of calcaneal osteomyelitis undergoing total or partial calcanectomy and intraoperative use of vancomycin powder showed no clinical benefit versus those that did not have the antibiotic powder applied.[38]

The use of cemented antibiotic beads can assist with stabilizing cortical structures by filling the dead space created after surgical debridement of the necrotic infected bone. Use of cemented antibiotic beads is inexpensive and can be tailored to specific organisms. Diabetic foot osteomyelitis can also be treated with biodegradable calcium sulfate beads impregnated with antibiotics for treatment of multidrug-resistant organisms in clinical circumstances that involve the following: poor circulation, polymicrobial growth, and associated renal and cardiac comorbidities.[39] Antibiotics used with calcium sulfate include colistin, meropenem, and vancomycin. Other studies have used antibiotic and antifungal agents including vancomycin, gentamicin, tobramycin, amphotericin B, and daptomycin (**Fig. 7**).

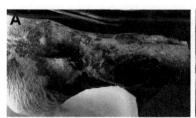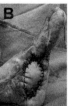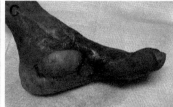

Fig. 6. Ulceration on the medial midfoot that had previously undergone bone resection and failed to heal with hemisoleus muscle flap and local tissue rearrangement (*A*). An island medial plantar artery perforator flap was performed to cover the midfoot osseous defect (*B, C*).

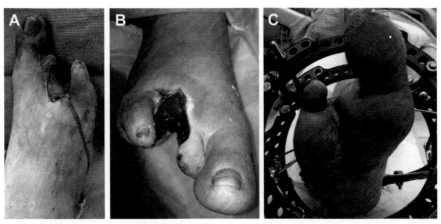

Fig. 7. Management of a soft tissue defect following open central ray amputation with nonbiodegradable drug delivery implant (*A*). Appearance of the surgical wound following removal of the cemented antibiotic block 6 weeks after implantation (*B*). Cleft defect managed with compression of forefoot with tensioned crossing olive wire fixation and wound closure with split-thickness skin graft (*C*).

Last, hyperbaric oxygen therapy has been used routinely as adjunctive outpatient treatment of patients with chronic osteomyelitis. Aerobic respiration can enhance bacteriocidic properties of some antibiotics, such as β-lactams, aminoglycosides, and fluroquinolones, by targeting O_2-depleted biofilms with hyperbaric oxygen treatment.[40,41] Aerobic respiration also provides an environment that stimulates angiogenesis and decreased edema of the soft tissue. Hyperbaric oxygen therapy is associated with decreased amputation rates and accelerated healing of nonischemic ulcerations. Although it is a useful adjuvant treatment, its consideration for being used should not delay operative treatment.

SUMMARY

Osteomyelitis is a limb-threatening diagnosis that requires a multidisciplinary approach for the best clinical outcome. An academic setting provides the treating physician and surgeon with the best diagnostic resources and allows for collaboration between the hospitalists, infection disease specialists, and vascular interventionists to optimize the patient for surgical debridement restoring the function to the affected limb; this requires advance planning and often involves staged reconstruction of the limb for the best surgical outcome. In addition, it is always important to remember that in certain clinical case scenarios, a proximal leg amputation is not a failed treatment of osteomyelitis. With proper recovery, rehabilitation, and lower extremity prosthesis, patients may return to their normal daily activities.

DISCLOSURE

Authors have nothing to disclose.

REFERENCES

1. Jhaveri VV, Sullivan C, Ward A, et al. More specialties, less problems: using collaborative competency between infectious disease, podiatry, and pathology

to improve the care of patients with diabetic foot osteomyelitis. J Am Podiatr Med Assoc 2021;20–178. https://doi.org/10.7547/20-178.

2. Lumbers M. Osteomyelitis, diabetic foot ulcers and the role of the community nurse. Br J Community Nurs 2021;26(Sup6):S6–9.

3. Ferrao P, Myerson MS, Schuberth JM, et al. Cement spacer as definitive management for postoperative ankle infection. Foot Ankle Int 2012;33(3):173–8.

4. Bach AW, Hansen ST Jr. Plates versus external fixation in severe open tibial shaft fractures. A randomized trial. Clin Orthop Relat Res 1989;(241):89–94.

5. Davidovitch RI, Elkataran R, Romo S, et al. Open reduction with internal fixation versus limited internal fixation and external fixation for high grade pilon fractures (OTA type 43C). Foot Ankle Int 2011;32(10):955–61.

6. Dalinka MK, Lally JF, Koniver G, et al. The radiology of osseous and articular infection. CRC Crit Rev Clin Radiol Nucl Med 1975;7(1):1–64.

7. Curtiss PH Jr. Some uncommon forms of osteomyelitis. Clin Orthop Relat Res 1973;(96):84–7.

8. El-Maghraby TA, Moustafa HM, Pauwels EK. Nuclear medicine methods for evaluation of skeletal infection among other diagnostic modalities. Q J Nucl Med Mol Imaging 2006;50(3):167–92.

9. Santiago Restrepo C, Gimenez CR, McCarthy K. Imaging of osteomyelitis and musculoskeletal soft tissue infections: current concepts. Rheum Dis Clin North Am 2003;29(1):89–109.

10. Vouillarmet J, Tordo J, Moret M, et al. 99mTc-white blood cell SPECT/CT to assess diabetic foot osteomyelitis remission: contribution of semi-quantitative scoring system. Nucl Med Commun 2021;42(7):713–8.

11. Dillon RS. Successful treatment of osteomyelitis and soft tissue infections in ischemic diabetic legs by local antibiotic injections and the end-diastolic pneumatic compression boot. Ann Surg 1986;204(6):643–9.

12. Gentry LO. Osteomyelitis: options for diagnosis and management. J Antimicrob Chemother 1988;21(Suppl C):115–31.

13. Lavery LA, Ahn J, Ryan EC, et al. What are the optimal cutoff values for ESR and CRP to Diagnose osteomyelitis in patients with diabetes-related foot infections? Clin Orthop Relat Res 2019;477(7):1594–602.

14. Vangaveti VN, Heyes O, Jhamb S, et al. Usefulness of procalcitonin in diagnosing diabetic foot osteomyelitis: a pilot study. Wounds 2021;33(7):192–6.

15. Soleimani Z, Amighi F, Vakili Z, et al. Diagnostic value of procalcitonin, erythrocyte sedimentation rate (ESR), quantitative C-reactive protein (CRP) and clinical findings associated with osteomyelitis in patients with diabetic foot. Hum Antibodies 2021;29(2):115–21.

16. Li X, Cheng Q, Du Z, et al. Microbiological concordance in the management of diabetic foot ulcer infections with osteomyelitis, on the basis of cultures of different specimens at a diabetic foot center in China. Diabetes Metab Syndr Obes 2021;14:1493–503.

17. Resnick D NG. Diagnosis of bone and joint disorders. 3rd edition. Philadelphia: WB Saunders; 1995.

18. Howard JB, McCracken GH Jr. The spectrum of group B streptococcal infections in infancy. Am J Dis Child 1974;128(6):815–8.

19. Kelly PJ. Osteomyelitis in the adult. Orthop Clin North Am 1975;6(4):983–9.

20. Andrianaki AM, Koutserimpas C, Kafetzakis A, et al. Diabetic foot infection and osteomyelitis. Are deep-tissue cultures necessary? Germs 2020;10(4):346–55.

21. Tardaguila-Garcia A, Sanz-Corbalán I, García-Morales E, et al. Diagnostic accuracy of bone culture versus biopsy in diabetic foot osteomyelitis. Adv Skin Wound Care 2021;34(4):204–8.

22. Lienard A, Hosny M, Jneid J, et al. Escherichia coli Isolated from diabetic foot osteomyelitis: clonal diversity, resistance profile, virulence potential, and genome adaptation. Microorganisms 2021;9(2):380.

23. Tardaguila-Garcia A, Sanz-Corbalán I, García-Alamino JM, et al. Medical versus surgical treatment for the management of diabetic foot osteomyelitis: a systematic review. J Clin Med 2021;10(6):1237.

24. Tardaguila-Garcia A, García-Álvarez Y, García-Morales E, et al. Long-term complications after surgical or medical treatment of predominantly forefoot diabetic foot osteomyelitis: 1 Year follow up. J Clin Med 2021;10(9):1943.

25. Lipsky BA, Uckay I. Treating diabetic foot osteomyelitis: a practical state-of-the-art update. Medicina (Kaunas) 2021;57(4).

26. Aragon-Sanchez J, Víquez-Molina G, López-Valverde ME, et al. Conservative surgery for diabetic foot osteomyelitis is not associated with longer Survival time without recurrence of foot ulcer when compared with amputation. Int J Low Extrem Wounds 2021. 15347346211009403.

27. Elmarsafi T, Pierre AJ, Wang K, et al. The vertical contour calcanectomy: an alternative surgical technique to the Conventional partial calcanectomy. J Foot Ankle Surg 2019;58(2):381–6.

28. Fisher TK, Armstrong DG. Partial calcanectomy in high-risk patients with diabetes: use and utility of a "hurricane" incisional approach. Eplasty 2010;10:e17.

29. Babiak I, Pędzisz P, Kulig M, et al. Comparison of bone preserving and radical surgical treatment in 32 cases of calcaneal osteomyelitis. J Bone Jt Infect 2016;1:10–6.

30. McCann MJ, Wells A. Calcaneal osteomyelitis: current treatment concepts. Int J Low Extrem Wounds 2020;19(3):230–5.

31. Baravarian B, Menendez MM, Weinheimer DJ, et al. Subtotal calcanectomy for the treatment of large heel ulceration and calcaneal osteomyelitis in the diabetic patient. J Foot Ankle Surg 1999;38(3):194–202.

32. Oliver NG, Steinberg JS, Powers K, et al. Lower extremity function following partial calcanectomy in high-risk limb salvage patients. J Diabetes Res 2015;2015:432164.

33. Smith DG, Stuck RM, Ketner L, et al. Partial calcanectomy for the treatment of large ulcerations of the heel and calcaneal osteomyelitis. An amputation of the back of the foot. J Bone Joint Surg Am 1992;74(4):571–6.

34. Brucato MP, Wachtler MF, Nasser EM. Osteomyelitis of the calcaneus with pathologic fracture. J Foot Ankle Surg 2019;58(3):591–5.

35. Folk JW, Starr AJ, Early JS. Early wound complications of operative treatment of calcaneus fractures: analysis of 190 fractures. J Orthop Trauma 1999;13(5):369–72.

36. Fox CM, Beem HM, Wiper J, et al. Muscle versus fasciocutaneous free flaps in heel reconstruction: systematic review and meta-analysis. J Reconstr Microsurg 2015;31(1):59–66.

37. Bibbo C, Siddiqui N, Fink J, et al. Wound coverage options for soft tissue defects following calcaneal fracture management (Operative/Surgical). Clin Podiatr Med Surg 2019;36(2):323–37.

38. Brodell JD Jr, Kozakiewicz LN, Hoffman SL, et al. Intraoperative site vancomycin powder Application in infected diabetic heel ulcers with calcaneal osteomyelitis. Foot Ankle Int 2021;42(3):356–62.

39. Patil P, Singh R, Agarwal A, et al. Diabetic foot ulcers and osteomyelitis: use of biodegradable calcium sulfate beads impregnated with antibiotics for treatment of multidrug-resistant organisms. Wounds 2021;33(3):70–6.

40. Kolpen M, Mousavi N, Sams T, et al. Reinforcement of the bactericidal effect of ciprofloxacin on Pseudomonas aeruginosa biofilm by hyperbaric oxygen treatment. Int J Antimicrob Agents 2016;47(2):163–7.

41. Dwyer DJ, Belenky PA, Yang JH, et al. Antibiotics induce redox-related physiological alterations as part of their lethality. Proc Natl Acad Sci U S A 2014;111(20): E2100–9.

Local Random Flaps for the Diabetic Foot

Shrunjay R. Patel, DPM, AACFAS*

KEYWORDS

- Diabetic foot • Neuropathy • Local random flap • Ulcer

KEY POINTS

- Diabetic foot and ankle wounds that fail to heal from local wound care therapy and offloading techniques, may require local skin flap to achieve wound closure.
- Patient must be optimized medically pre-operatively to achieve successful outcomes after local skin flap appJcation.
- Careful intraoperative manipulation of soft tissue will minimize trauma to the flap and increase flap survival.
- Appropriate non-weight bearing and offloading is a must after local flap application.

INTRODUCTION

With the rise in prevalence of diabetes worldwide, there has been a corresponding increase in the occurrence of diabetic foot wounds.[1–7] Diabetic foot wounds may occur due to a triad of vasculopathy, neuropathy, and foot deformity.[8] Peripheral sensory and motor neuropathy can lead to an insensate foot and abnormal foot function, which when combined with repetitive trauma during gait may cause ulceration.[9] Foot and ankle wounds that are recalcitrant to local wound care modalities and traditional off-loading techniques may require surgical wound closure and within the soft tissue reconstructive pyramid, local random skin flaps represent an advanced option.[10]

PREOPERATIVE CONSIDERATIONS

Infection, uncontrolled diabetes mellitus, peripheral vascular disease, poor nutrition, and biomechanical abnormalities should be considered before performing a local flap closure. Infection and biofilm must be thoroughly debrided from the wound base before application of local random flaps. Recent studies show that glycosylated hemoglobin levels higher than 8% are associated with poor surgical outcomes; therefore, an endocrinology consultation may be warranted before surgery.[11] Malnutrition is

Division of Vascular Surgery, Department of Surgery, University of North Carolina, Chapel Hill, NC, USA
* 130 Annabelle Branch Lane, Apex, NC 27523.
E-mail address: shrunjay@gmail.com

Clin Podiatr Med Surg 39 (2022) 321–330
https://doi.org/10.1016/j.cpm.2021.11.004

an independent risk factor associated with delayed wound healing and also should be optimized.[12] Vascular insufficiency is detrimental to local skin flap survival. A vascular surgery consultation should be considered for ankle brachial index of less than 0.7, toe pressures of less than 30 mm Hg, or transcutaneous oxygen tension levels of less than 30 mm Hg.[13] Biomechanical abnormalities such as gastrocnemius or gastrocnemius-soleal equinus, plantarflexed metatarsals, Charcot neuroarthropathy with rocker bottom deformity, calcaneal gait, and hammertoe contractures also should be addressed either before or during the same surgical encounter as the local random flap.[8,14]

Local random flaps are extremely useful in achieving wound closure at the plantar aspect of the foot.[15] They include epidermis, dermis, and subcutaneous tissue, and also may include underlying fascia and muscle, therefore can match the shock-absorbing ability of the plantar tissues to combat sheer forces.[16,17] Indications for local random flaps of the foot include wounds with exposed vital structures (bone, hardware, joint, tendons, neurovascular bundle), wounds on weight-bearing surfaces, and wounds requiring reduction of scar from multiple previous wounds or surgical wounds. Contraindications include infection or inadequate wound bed preparation, peripheral vascular disease that impairs perfusion to the foot and cannot be corrected, lack of tissue expansibility or durability at the donor site, large soft tissue defects, poor patient compliance, or inability to remain non–weight bearing.

Local random flaps are most classified based on the design and the method of transfer: advancement, rotation, transposition. Pre-planning of flap design is very important, as the surgeon may be able to resect the underlying osteomyelitis or osseous deformity from the same incision, which would allow increased tissue laxity, and thus permit easier tissue transfer and avoid extrasurgical incisions.[8] Once the flap is designed and marked out, the flap should be raised below the subdermal plexus from the opposite edge of healthy tissue toward the wound defect, as the tissue planes are better defined in donor tissue compared with the chronic wound. When raising the flap at the plantar aspect of the foot, the defined ligaments connecting the plantar fascia to the plantar fat pad are carefully released, and the full thickness flap is raised while preserving the perforating vessels as much as possible.

It is also recommended that undermining of the flap should be kept to a minimum to avoid any iatrogenic injury to the subdermal plexus, which can cause partial or complete necrosis of the flap. Careful atraumatic meticulous dissection under loupe magnification is recommended. Retraction should be used only when needed, and gentle tissue handling should be implemented to avoid inadvertent tissue injury. It is equally important to achieve hemostasis before the wound closure because this can lead to hematoma formation, which can affect flap viability. Furthermore, hematoma can become a nidus for infection.[18] Therefore, flap dissection under tourniquet utilization and bipolar electrocautery for cauterizing any blood vessels with minimal deep sutures to avoid ischemia deep to the flap is highly recommended.[18]

INTRAOPERATIVE CONSIDERATIONS

Meticulous dissection and gentle tissue handling techniques increase chances of flap survival. Excessive retraction and significant undermining of the tissue around the flap tissue should be avoided. Incisions should be made perpendicular to the skin without skiving and separating the layers of the skin. Care should be taken not to kink or twist the flaps while transferring. If the flap turns white or cyanotic while transferring, then the flap should be placed back in its anatomic location and "delayed" for 4 to 7 days. A delayed phenomenon causes vasodilation of the existing blood vessels in the flap, which increases vascularity within the flap and increases the rate of flap survival.[19] Using fluorescein dye is another very useful way of checking vascularity within the flap.[20] Other causes of flap failure include infection, tight bandages, shear forces, hematoma/seroma, edema, and venous congestion. Care should be taken to achieve complete hemostasis before the application of bandages, and these should be applied lightly without excessive compression. The affected extremity should be elevated to decrease edema. Preoperative and postoperative antibiotic course may be considered to prevent infection.

ADVANCEMENT FLAP

Surgical technique in performing an advancement flap involves advancing the tissue in one single direction. Typically, advancement flaps are used to cover metatarsal head defects at the plantar or medial forefoot areas but also can be used in the midfoot area. Perfusion to the advancement flap comes from the subdermal plexus and local perforators; therefore, undermining into the flap should be avoided to prevent flap necrosis. As the distance to the leading edge from the feeding artery or arteriole increases, oxygenated blood reaching the leading edge decreases. There are several variations

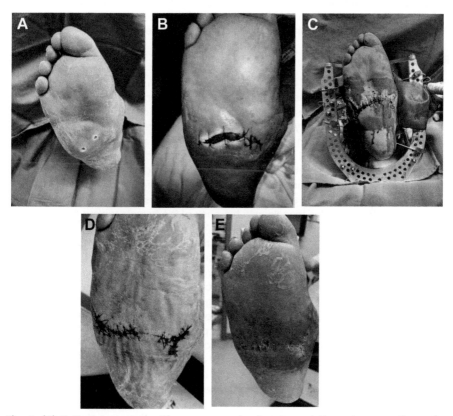

Fig. 1. (*A*) Patient presented with open wounds, abscess, and Charcot neuroarthropathy with rocker bottom deformity. (*B*) Initial surgical incision and drainage was performed with retention sutures. (*C*) Patient was brought back to the operating room for revision incision and drainage and plantar ostectomy. Double advancement flap was performed and surgical off-loading was achieved with the application of a circular external fixation device. (*D*) Patient returned to the operating room for the external fixation removal. (*E*) Patient healed completely at the final postoperative visit.

of the advancement flap, such as single advancement, double advancement (**Fig. 1**), V-Y, and double V-Y.

The single advancement flap is created by making 2 parallel incisions away from the defect and the flap is harvested below the subdermal plexus and advanced toward the defect along the single axis to close the wound. The Burrow triangles are resected away from the flap. Back cuts also can be made into the base of the flap but it is not recommended, as it can compromise the subdermal plexus and vascularity of the flap. Approximately up to 1 to 2 cm of the defect at the plantar aspect of the foot can be covered with this type of the flap.[8] If the defect is 3 to 4 cm long, or tension on the leading edge after single advancement flap, a double advancement flap on the opposite site of the wound can be harvested for wound closure.[8]

The V-Y flap is a type of an island flap. The length of the "V" is approximately 2 to 3 times the base of the flap.[21,22] The incision is made perpendicular through the skin down to the subcutaneous tissue level without undermining it. As the flap is advanced toward the defect, skin on the opposite site of the apex of the flap is sutured together so the shape goes from a "V" to a "Y." Such flaps are useful in areas in the forefoot for metatarsal head ulcerations or midfoot ulcerations.[21,22] Up to 1 to 2 cm of the wound defect can be covered with a V-Y flap.[22] If the defect is large, a double V-Y flap from the opposite side of the wound can be raised to cover the defect.

ROTATION FLAPS

Rotation flaps rotate or pivot around a fixed point through an arc of rotation to cover the defect.[23] A benefit of these flaps over an advancement flap is that the tension is shared across larger donor tissue, and the design can be used to cover larger defects as well.[23] Rotation flaps are typically used to cover defects in the midfoot or hindfoot/malleolar areas.[24–26] Rotation flaps can be of a random or an axial pattern, depending on the level of dissection and if a known artery is dissected along with flap dissection. For example, the medial plantar artery can be incorporated when the rotational flap is harvested to cover the forefoot, midfoot, and hindfoot defects (**Fig. 2**).

A single rotation flap is the simplest form of rotation flaps. First, the wound defect is converted into an isosceles triangle with the apex of the triangle toward the donor site and with an apex angle of no more than 30°.[27] An incision is then made in the form of a semicircle or arc from the superior aspect of the wound base. The incision length is approximately 4 to 5 times the width of the base of the triangular defect. Tissue is then rotated around a fixed pivot point toward the wound defect. The pivot point is close to the apex of the wound defect. Typically, a back cut is required to effectively move the tissue without significant tension along the leading edge.[27] One can perform a back cut in the flap or away from the flap. If the back cut is performed into the flap, it can compromise circulation. On the other hand, if the back cut is performed away from the flap, a Burrow triangle is excised and tension-free closure is achieved.[27]

A double rotation flap is another variation of a single classic rotation flap in which a second flap is raised from the opposite side of the isosceles triangle, and tissue is moved toward the defect with the same diameter and same pivot point as the single rotation flap. Frequently, the donor tissue is rotated, a secondary donor wound defect arises that can be addressed with the application of a split-thickness skin graft or acellular dermal replacement.

TRANSPOSITION FLAPS

Transposition flaps are a combination of the rotation and advancement flaps. These flaps typically have narrower bases than a rotational flap. To cover the same size of

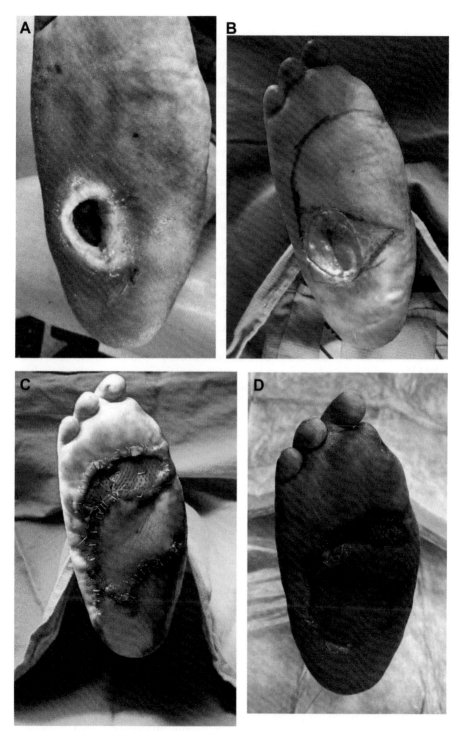

Fig. 2. (*A*) Patient presented with a nonhealing wound for several years with failed conservative therapy. (*B*) Staged surgical debridements and biopsy were performed without any

wound defect, transposition flaps require less tissue mobilization compared with a rotation flap; however, unlike rotation flaps, skin grafts may be required to cover the secondary defect caused by the transposition flap. Transposition flaps can be used to cover a large area of wound defect in the midfoot, hindfoot, heel, and malleoli.[8,28,29] A simple transpositional flap is created first by excising the original wound defect into a square or rectangle, then the adjacent tissue of same width and length is raised below the subdermal plexus and pivoted around a fixed point to cover the original defect. It is preferable to have a known perforator or artery at the base.[8] One of the biggest disadvantages of such flaps is that it leaves a secondary defect that needs to be covered by skin grafting. These flaps are typically used to cover wound defects of metatarsal heads, midfoot, heel, medial, or lateral malleoli wounds.[8] Many variations of the transpositional flap exist and can be used to cover defects in the foot, including monolobed or bilobed flap, simple transpositional flap (**Fig. 3**), Z-plasty (single or multiple), Limberg flap, and double-Z-rhomboid flap.

Single lobe flaps, also known as Schrudde flaps or slide-swing plasty, are useful in covering small circular, oval or semicircular defects. Typically, they are used after excising a mucoid cyst, intractable porokeratosis, or an ulcer of the digit or metatarsal head.[30] Once the wound is excised in the shape of a circle or oval, a semi-oval or lobe-shaped incision at 90° to the base of the original defect is created, with the diameter of the flap approximately 75% of the size of the original defect and the length-to-width ratio of close to 1:1.[31] The flap is then raised below the subdermal plexus and rotated into the defect and the secondary defect is closed primarily. If there is tension on the flap, edges away from the flap can be undermined as needed. Variations of this flap also exist in which the axis of the lobe is approximately 45 to 60° to the base of the defect.[32]

Bilobed flaps consist of 2-lobe flaps of progressively decreasing size with an angle of 90° between the flaps with a shared blood supply.[33] This flap is ideal for defects smaller than 1.5 cm in diameter. The size of the first lobe is typically 75% of the original defect and the second lobe is typically 50% of the size of the secondary defect. Although variation of the angles and the size exist in the literature, the goal is that the primary and secondary defect is closed without need for skin grafting. This flap is useful when larger tissue needs to be mobilized and the defect cannot be covered by a monolobed flap. Typically, bilobed flap closure is used to cover forefoot wounds, including wounds on toes, and plantar and dorsal metatarsal heads.[32]

The Z-plasty technique is extremely beneficial in elongating and redirecting scar tissue.[33] The central arm of the "Z" is in the direction in which the scar or tissue needs to be lengthened.[33] Two parallel diagonal incisions are then made approximately 45 to 60° from the end of the central arm. The 2 arms of the Z-plasty are then dissected below the subdermal plexus and transposed over and sutured at midpoint first on the outside and then at the central arm. Typically, a 30° angle of the triangle would increase the length by only 25%, while a 75° angle would allow the length to increase by 100%.[20] However, the higher the angle close to 90°, the more difficult the closure. Multiple Z-plasties can often be used to preserve vascularity as opposed to a single large Z-plasty with wide angles and large arms.[20]

---

evidence of osteomyelitis. (*C*) Plantar exostectomy combined with a single fasciocutaneous rotation flap based on the medial plantar artery flap was harvested and inset in the recipient site. The donor site was covered with an autogenous split-thickness skin graft. (*D*) The patient healed well at the final postoperative follow-up.

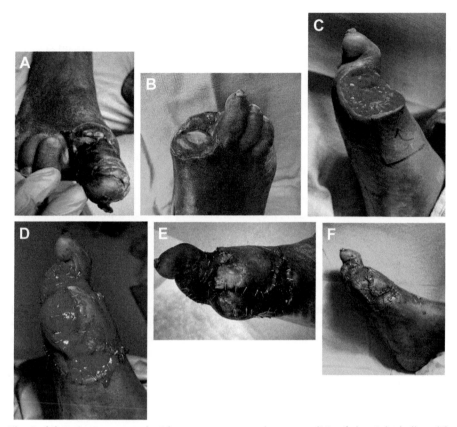

Fig. 3. (*A*) Patient presented with gas gangrene and osteomyelitis of the right hallux. (*B*) Staged hallux amputation was performed with debridement of the infected soft tissue. (*C*) After angioplasty of the anterior tibial artery, the patient was brought back to the operating room for further surgical debridement, partial first metatarsal head resection, and coverage of the exposed bone. (*D*) A single transposition flap was harvested dorsally and plantar tissue was advanced and inset to cover the first metatarsal bone. The donor site was covered with a bilayer meshed collagen acellular dermal replacement. (*E*) Patient flap and graft healing well postoperatively. (*F*) Patient was brought back to operating room for surgical debridement of the wound and application of autogenous split-thickness skin graft.

Many variations of Z-plasty exist, and it is very useful in digital surgery such as desyndactylization of toes, revisional hammertoe surgery, or hyperextension deformity at the metatarsal phalangeal joint.[20]

The Limberg or rhomboid flap is a versatile flap in the reconstruction of diabetic foot wounds. The original defect is initially converted into a rhombus-shaped parallelogram with sides of equal length and angles of 60° and 120° on the opposite sides. Four possible choices for flap design exist. The flap that lies within the greatest amount of skin laxity and the flap that has direct inline blood flow is typically chosen. If there is any tension on the leading edge of the flap, then a second flap should be raised on the diagonal side of the wound defect to allow for inflow from the opposite side. The rhomboid flap is useful in covering defects at the medial aspect of the first or fifth metatarsals, plantar midfoot, and medial or lateral malleolus.

A double Z-rhomboid flap is a useful flap in treating wound defects of the plantar midfoot or metatarsal head area.[20] In this flap, the wound defect is excised in the shape of a rhomboid, and 2 Z-plasties are then created on the opposite ends of the rhomboid defect. The 4 arms of the double Z-plasties are then transposed over, and the wound is closed primarily without needing a skin graft.

POSTOPERATIVE CARE

Close observation and follow-up is required after performing local random flaps in the foot and ankle regions of diabetic patients. Patients should remain non–weight bearing with well-padded posterior splints or via circular external fixations to avoid any direct pressure against the flap. If there is concern of vascularity of the flap, the flap can be checked by sticking with an 18-gauge needle. If bright red blood is noted, that would mean adequate arterial perfusion. On other hand, if delayed bleeding is noted, that would indicate an arterial spasm. If cyanotic bleeding is noted, it would mean venous congestion. Arterial spasms can be improved by removing sutures and relieving tension on the pedicle, whereas venous congestion can be improved by using medicinal leeches.[34]

SUMMARY

Reconstruction of wounds in the diabetic foot and ankle can be achieved by several different local random flap techniques. Improper flap selection, inadequate surgical debridement, presence of infection, traumatic surgical techniques, and flap closure under tension can lead to flap failure. Patients should be placed on a strict non–weight-bearing postoperative protocol with elevation of the affected extremity to prevent venous congestion. When executed correctly with careful patient selection, local random flaps for the diabetic foot and ankle can be an invaluable surgical tool.

CLINICS CARE POINTS

- Selection of the type of local random flap depends on the location of the wound. Selecting inappropriate flap can lead to excess tension on the flap which can lead to flap failure.
- Rotation flaps and transposition flaps must be dissected below subdermal plexus. Whereas, subdermal plexus should be preserved for advancement flap.
- If flap turns white or cyanotic while harvesting, flap transposition should be delayed for 4-7 days.

REFERENCES

1. Coexisting conditions and complications. Centers for Disease Control and Prevention; 2020. Available at: https://www.cdc.gov/diabetes/data/statistics-report/coexisting-conditions-complications.html. Accessed August 12, 2021.
2. Yazdanpanah L, Nasiri M, Adarvishi S. Literature review on the management of diabetic foot ulcer. World J Diabetes 2015;6(1):37. https://doi.org/10.4239/wjd.v6.i1.37.
3. Gershater MA, Löndahl M, Nyberg P, et al. Complexity of factors related to outcome of neuropathic and neuroischaemic/ischaemic diabetic foot ulcers: a cohort study. Diabeologia 2008;52(3):398–407. https://doi.org/10.1007/s00125-008-1226-2.

4. Ikura K, Hanai K, Oka S, et al. Brachial-ankle pulse wave velocity, but not ankle-brachial index, predicts all-cause mortality in patients with diabetes after lower extremity amputation. J Diabetes Invest 2016;8(2):250–3. https://doi.org/10.1111/jdi.12554.

5. Martins-Mendes D, Monteiro-Soares M, Boyko EJ, et al. The independent contribution of diabetic foot ulcer on lower extremity amputation and mortality risk. J Diabetes its Complications 2014;28(5):632–8. https://doi.org/10.1016/j.jdiacomp.2014.04.011.

6. Yotsu RR, Pham NM, Oe M, et al. Comparison of characteristics and healing course of diabetic foot ulcers by etiological classification: neuropathic, ischemic, and neuro-ischemic type. J Diabetes Complications 2014;28(4):528–35. https://doi.org/10.1016/j.jdiacomp.2014.03.013.

7. McEwen LN, Ylitalo KR, Herman WH, et al. Prevalence and risk factors for diabetes-related foot complications in translating research into action for diabetes (triad). J Diabetes Complications 2013;27(6):588–92. https://doi.org/10.1016/j.jdiacomp.2013.08.003.

8. Clemens M, Attinger C. Functional reconstruction of the diabetic foot. Semin Plast Surg 2010;24(01):043–56. https://doi.org/10.1055/s-0030-1253239.

9. Hicks CW, Selvin E. Epidemiology of peripheral neuropathy and lower extremity disease in diabetes. Curr Diab Rep 2019;19(10):86. https://doi.org/10.1007/s11892-019-1212-8.

10. Capobianco CM, Stapleton JJ, Zgonis T. Soft tissue reconstruction pyramid in the diabetic foot. Foot Ankle Spec 2010;3(5):241–8. https://doi.org/10.1177/1938640010375113.

11. Underwood P, Askari R, Hurwitz S, et al. Response to comment on Underwood et al. Preoperative A1C and clinical outcomes in patients with diabetes undergoing major noncardiac surgical procedures. Diabetes Care 2014;37:611–616. Diabetes Care 2014;37(8):e191. https://doi.org/10.2337/dc14-0738.

12. Sajid N, Miyan Z, Zaidi SI, et al. Protein requirement and its intake in subjects with diabetic foot ulcers at a tertiary care hospital. Pakistan J Med Sci 2018;34(4):886–90. https://doi.org/10.12669/pjms.344.15399.

13. Tay WL, Lo ZJ, Hong Q, et al. Toe pressure in predicting diabetic foot ulcer healing: a systematic review and meta-analysis. Ann Vasc Surg 2019;60:371–8. https://doi.org/10.1016/j.avsg.2019.04.011.

14. Lázaro-Martínez JL, Aragón-Sánchez J, Álvaro-Afonso FJ, et al. The best way to reduce reulcerations. Int J Lower Extrem Wounds 2014;13(4):294–319. https://doi.org/10.1177/1534734614549417.

15. Zgonis T, Stapleton JJ, Roukis TS. Advanced plastic surgery techniques for soft tissue coverage of the diabetic foot. Clin Podiatric Med Surg 2007;24(3):547–68. https://doi.org/10.1016/j.cpm.2007.03.002.

16. Oh SJ, Moon M, Cha J, et al. Weight-bearing plantar reconstruction using versatile medial plantar sensate flap. J Plast Reconstr Aesthet Surg 2011;64(2):248–54. https://doi.org/10.1016/j.bjps.2010.04.013.

17. Blume PA, Paragas LK, Sumpio BE, et al. Single-stage surgical treatment of noninfected diabetic foot ulcers. Plast Reconstr Surg 2002;109(2):601–9. https://doi.org/10.1097/00006534-200202000-00029.

18. Jolly GP, Zgonis T, Blume P. Soft tissue reconstruction of the diabetic foot. Clin Podiatric Med Surg 2003;20(4):757–81. https://doi.org/10.1016/s0891-8422(03)00072-7.

19. Tosun Z, Özkan A, Karaçor Z, et al. Delaying the reverse sural flap provides predictable results for complicated wounds in diabetic foot. Ann Plast Surg 2005; 55(2):169–73. https://doi.org/10.1097/01.sap.0000170530.51470.1a.

20. Zgonis T. Surgical reconstruction of the diabetic foot and ankle. Philadelphia, PA: Wolters Kluwer; 2018.

21. Roukis TS, Schweinberger MH, Schade VL, et al. Fasciocutaneous advancement flap coverage of soft tissue defects of the foot in the patient at high risk. J Foot Ankle Surg 2010;49(1):71–4. https://doi.org/10.1053/j.jfas.2009.04.006.

22. Colen LB, Replogle SL, Mathes SJ. The V-Y plantar flap for reconstruction of the forefoot. Plast Reconstr Surg 1988;81(2):220–7. https://doi.org/10.1097/00006534-198802000-00014.

23. Scaglioni MF, Rittirsch D, Giovanoli P. Reconstruction of the heel, middle foot sole, and plantar forefoot with the medial plantar artery perforator flap. Plast Reconstr Surg 2018;141(1):200–8. https://doi.org/10.1097/prs.0000000000003975.

24. Boffeli TJ, Collier RC. Near total calcanectomy with rotational flap closure of large decubitus heel ulcerations complicated by calcaneal osteomyelitis. J Foot Ankle Surg 2013;52(1):107–12. https://doi.org/10.1053/j.jfas.2012.06.018.

25. Boffeli TJ, Reinking R. Plantar rotational flap technique for panmetatarsal head resection and transmetatarsal amputation: a revision approach for second metatarsal head transfer ulcers in patients with previous partial first ray amputation. J Foot Ankle Surg 2014;53(1):96–100. https://doi.org/10.1053/j.jfas.2013.06.011.

26. Boffeli TJ, Peterson MC. Rotational flap closure of first and fifth metatarsal head plantar ulcers: adjunctive procedure when performing first or fifth ray amputation. J Foot Ankle Surg 2013;52(2):263–70. https://doi.org/10.1053/j.jfas.2012.10.020.

27. Patel KG, Sykes JM. Concepts in local flap design and classification. Oper Tech Otolaryngol Head Neck Surg 2011;22(1):13–23. https://doi.org/10.1016/j.otot.2010.09.002.

28. Congdon GC, Altman MI, Aldridge J. A comparison of transpositional neurovascular skin flaps for reconstruction of diabetic heel ulcerations. J Foot Surg 1988; 27:127–9.

29. Park EY, Elliott ED, Giacopelli JA, et al. The use of transpositional skin flaps in closing plantar defects: a case report. J Foot Ankle Surg 1997;36(4):315–21. https://doi.org/10.1016/s1067-2516(97)80080-4.

30. Dockery GL. Single-lobe rotation flaps. J Am Podiatric Med Assoc 1995;85(1): 36–40. https://doi.org/10.7547/87507315-85-1-36.

31. Boffeli TJ, Hyllengren SB. Unilobed rotational flap for plantar hallux interphalangeal joint ulceration complicated by osteomyelitis. J Foot Ankle Surg 2015; 54(6):1166–71. https://doi.org/10.1053/j.jfas.2014.12.023.

32. Bouch RT, Christensen JC, Hale DS. Unilobed and bilobed skin flaps. Detailed surgical technique for plantar lesions. J Am Podiatric Med Assoc 1995;85(1): 41–8. https://doi.org/10.7547/87507315-85-1-41.

33. Chang TJ, Stanifer EG, Jimenez AL. Plastic repair techniques: skin plasties and local flaps 1993. Available at: http://www.podiatryinstitute.com/pdfs/Update_1993/1993_31.pdf. Accessed August 1, 2021.

34. Jose M, Varghese J, Babu A. Salvage of venous congestion using medicinal leeches for traumatic nasal flap. J Maxillofacial Oral Surg 2013;14(S1):251–4. https://doi.org/10.1007/s12663-012-0468-1.

Surgical Considerations for the Acute and Chronic Charcot Neuroarthropathy of the Foot and Ankle

Check for updates

Alan C. Stuto, DPM[a],*, John J. Stapleton, DPM[b,c]

KEYWORDS

- Diabetic Charcot neuroarthopathy • Foot • Ankle • Trauma • Diabetic neuropathy

KEY POINTS

- Charcot neuroarthropathy (CN) is a progressive and destructive process that is characterized by acute fractures, dislocations, and joint destruction that will lead to foot and/or ankle deformities.
- Accurate diagnosis can be a difficult challenge in the acute/subacute stage of CN for the treating physician.
- Evolving surgical techniques have focused on increasing stability of fixation primarily by extending hardware proximally and distally into areas where the bone is not fragmented by the CN process.

INTRODUCTION

Depending on the clinical scenario, acute versus chronic Charcot neuroarthropathy (CN) should be managed independently with similar guiding principles. A wide array of surgical procedures can be used and should be tailored to each individual case, including soft tissue and/or bone debridement, biopsy, ostectomy, osteotomies, arthrodesis, allogenic and autogenous bone grafting, osseous shortening via tarsal bone resection or talectomy, open reduction internal fixation, multiplanar circular external fixation, equinus correction, tendon balancing procedures, plastic surgical techniques, and amputation.[1] This review article focuses on the surgical management of acute and chronic CN with case presentations.

---

[a] LVPG Orthopedics and Sports Medicine, Lehigh Valley Health Network, 2597 Schoenersville Road, Suite 100, Bethlehem, PA 18017, USA; [b] Division of Podiatric Surgery, LVPG Orthopedics and Sports Medicine, Lehigh Valley Health Network, 250 South Cedar Crest Boulevard, Suite 110, Allentown, PA 18103, USA; [c] Penn State College of Medicine, 500 University Drive, Hershey, PA 17033, USA
* Corresponding author.
E-mail address: alan.stuto@lvhn.org

Clin Podiatr Med Surg 39 (2022) 331–341
https://doi.org/10.1016/j.cpm.2021.11.005

PREOPERATIVE ASSESSMENT

Accurate diagnosis can be a difficult challenge in the acute/subacute stage of CN for the treating physician. The diagnosis of acute CN before radiographic findings is primarily clinical, requiring a high index of suspicion. The presentation is often confused with gouty arthropathy, deep venous thrombosis, and cellulitis. CN should be considered in diabetic patients with peripheral neuropathy who present with lower-extremity edema, erythema, and increased skin temperature, with or without ulceration. Pain may or may not be present in this patient population. Deformity may also not be present during the initial onset of this condition. In early acute CN, radiographic abnormalities may be subtle or absent, whereas diagnosis of chronic CN is easier, as it presents with recognizable foot and/or ankle deformities and obvious radiographic findings. Ulceration with or without infection is commonly encountered as a result of these chronic osseous deformities.

The initial workup of CN should involve radiographs to determine whether there are any osseous abnormalities. The radiographs help guide treatment and are used in addition to the clinical examination in staging the disease process. Early diagnostic findings on plain films are typically nonspecific or minimal. For this reason, serial radiographs over a 2- to 4-week period may be helpful in the suspected early acute phase of CN to establish or rule out the diagnosis, including contralateral lower-extremity views for comparison when needed. As the disease progresses, radiographic findings can include fractures usually with associated joint subluxation and/or dislocation, osseous fragmentation, sclerotic avascular bone, periosteal reaction, and/or heterotopic bone formation.

Advanced imaging can be helpful as an adjunctive tool, including MRI, computed tomography (CT) scan, and nuclear medicine imaging. MRI is sensitive for early detection of CN. It is useful when radiographs are inconclusive or negative and clinical suspicion remains high. In addition, MRI with and without contrast may be helpful to differentiate noninfected from an infected bone pathologic condition and to evaluate for deep infection/abscess formation. The presence of a sinus tract, replacement of soft tissue fat, and fluid collection on the contrast-enhanced MRI favors osteomyelitis over CN. Diffuse marrow involvement on MRI is frequently observed in the setting of CN and rarely with infection.[2] Radionucleotide bone scan, labeled white blood cell scan, and sulfur colloid are other tests that can be useful in discerning between CN and osteomyelitis but are not always specific. CT scan is useful for establishing a 3-dimensional view of the deformity and for surgical planning.

Additional diagnostic interventional procedures that can be useful in certain clinical scenarios to establish a diagnosis include synovial biopsy and bone biopsy/culture. Invasive techniques are typically reserved if other diagnostic modalities are inconclusive, concern for infection is present, and/or to rule out other neoplastic tumors if suspected. Synovial biopsy may reveal small fragments of bone and cartilage debris embedded in the synovium because of destruction of the joints, which is a finding that is suggestive of CN.

The surgeon cannot disregard the multiple comorbidities that are often present with patients who are diagnosed with CN. A multidisciplinary team is required to care for these patients that may include internal medicine, endocrinology, vascular surgery, cardiology, nephrology, infectious disease, and other specialists as needed. Optimization of blood sugars is vital to promote wound healing and reduce risk of postoperative infection. Medical optimization through one's primary care provider and medicine team is imperative as well. Patients with peripheral arterial disease may need vascular surgical intervention before definitive foot/ankle surgical intervention.

Nephrology may be needed especially with patients that are dialysis dependent. Infectious disease consultation may also be needed to coordinate care among patients with deep infections and/or concomitant osteomyelitis. Also, patients that have smoking, drug, and/or alcohol dependency will require ancillary services to establish cessation programs.

SURGICAL INTERVENTION FOR THE ACUTE AND CHRONIC CHARCOT NEUROARTHROPATHY

During the acute phase of CN, surgery may be considered in 2 clinical scenarios: (1) an unstable deformity usually as a result of a severe dislocation that will lead to soft tissue necrosis, and (2) a septic acute CN joint. Although controversial to perform surgery during the acute phase based on multiple experts and investigators, it is sometimes indicated to prevent further morbidity.[3–8] Surgical procedures are ultimately chosen depending on each clinical scenario. During the acute CN without infection but soft tissue jeopardy, goals of surgery will include stabilization of the deformity through either temporary reduction with external fixation or gradual correction of the deformity with circular external fixation and delayed osseous reconstruction/joint arthrodesis or one-stage osseous reconstruction/primary joint arthrodesis with internal and/or external fixation (**Fig. 1**).

During the acute CN with infection, this would typically be performed in a staged fashion with the focus of the first stage to eradicate infection before definitive osseous reconstruction. The first stage would include removal of all nonviable infected bone and/or soft tissue (which may need multiple surgical debridement procedures), along with obtaining intraoperative soft tissue/bone cultures and bone biopsy to help guide antibiotic management. Temporary spanning external fixators could be used during this stage to provide osseous stability while protecting the soft tissue envelope until definitive osseous reconstruction/joint arthrodesis can be performed. Often, external fixators are later modified in future staged procedures to avoid internal fixation given the infectious process that needs to be managed.

Ultimately, if surgery can be avoided during the acute phase of CN, it is usually preferable. Serial splinting and/or casting is favored to immobilize the extremity, reduce edema, and prevent further deformity. Once the acute phase subsides, which can take approximately 3 months or longer, the deformity should be reassessed to determine if nonoperative management can be considered. One must discern if the extremity can be braced adequately and if the patient can resume ambulation without ulceration. If the deformity is not amenable to conservative treatments, then deformity correction can be performed usually through osteotomies and/or joint arthrodesis with internal and/or external fixation. High consideration is also given to the extensive follow-up and ultimate duration of circular external fixation application when used early to stabilize a deformity or to gradually correct an acute CN deformity with the understanding that further reconstructive procedures will likely need to be performed. This extended period of time in a circular external fixator is a challenge for the patient both mentally and physically. Complications, such as pin/wire tract infections, breakage, osteomyelitis, and additional fractures, may increase the duration of the external fixator that is placed. Other complications to consider when operating on an acute CN is the increased hematoma formation that is present from the acute process of the condition itself, wound complications secondary to severe edema, and postoperative infections. In addition, operating on an acute CN often does not allow for sufficient time to medically optimize the patient with uncontrolled diabetes.

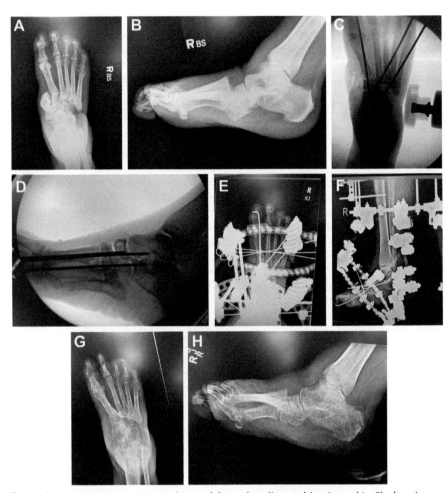

Fig. 1. Preoperative anteroposterior and lateral radiographic views (*A, B*) showing an acute CN with a Lisfranc fracture dislocation. Tension on the skin medially was leading to tissue necrosis. Acute surgical intervention was performed with a primary medial column arthrodesis (*C, D*) and application of a multiplanar circular external fixation (*E, F*). Final radiographic views demonstrate a stable medial column arthrodesis free of ulceration (*G, H*). Patient was ambulating 9 months postoperatively with diabetic shoes and custom inlays.

During the chronic phase of CN, surgery should be considered when conservative treatment fails or is not a viable treatment option. Indications for surgery include foot and ankle deformities that cannot be braced, deformities that do not allow for functional ambulation, and deformities that cause ulceration with or without infection (**Fig. 2**).[9] Osseous procedures during this phase can include ostectomy, osteotomies, bone resection, and arthrodesis procedures. Adjunctive soft tissue procedures to achieve tendon balancing can be performed through tendon transfers, tenotomies, percutaneous tendo-Achilles lengthening, and/or gastrocnemius recession when indicated.[10,11] Soft tissue coverage must be considered in addition to osseous reconstruction when ulceration and soft tissue loss are present.

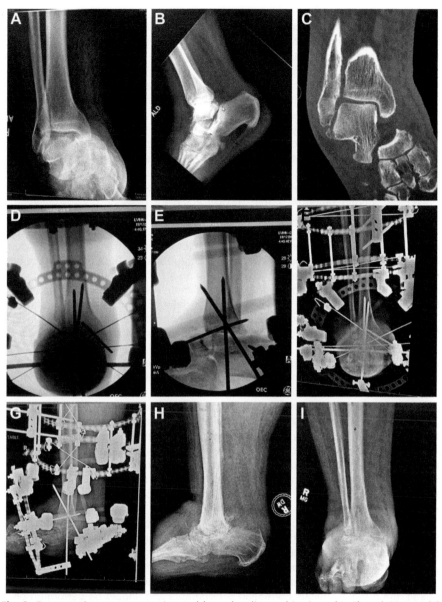

Fig. 2. Preoperative anteroposterior and lateral radiographic views (*A*, *B*) and CT scan (*C*) showing a right CN involving a talonavicular fracture/dislocation and a peritalar ankle/hind-foot varus deformity that was not amenable to bracing. Patient underwent a talectomy, ti-biocalcaneal arthrodesis with autogenous bone graft from the resected distal fibula (*D*, *E*), and application of a multiplanar circular external fixation (*F*, *G*). Final radiographic views at 7 months postoperatively demonstrating a successful tibiocalcaneal arthrodesis (*H*, *I*). Patient was ambulating with custom-made diabetic shoes and double upright brace to the right lower extremity.

If a wound is present that is clinically stable-appearing or free of infection, consideration can be made to close the ulceration primarily with a local flap after osseous resection and deformity correction is performed. Other considerations for wound closure that can be used are pedicle/perforator flaps, autogenous split-thickness skin grafts, or free tissue transfer. Often in the diabetic patient population, though, free tissue transfer can be challenging given the presence of underlying calcified vessels. For this reason, attempts are usually made to try to achieve soft tissue coverage with local flaps and pedicle/perforator flaps. In certain clinical scenarios, negative pressure wound therapy may be used with delayed soft tissue closure.

Ostectomy procedures should only be considered for chronic stable midfoot deformities and rocker-bottom deformities that are leading to soft tissue compromise. The surgeon must be aware that ostectomies may lead to further midfoot instability and collapse that could lead to failure. For this reason, it is important to perform ostectomy procedures among deformities that display sufficient osseous consolidation and remodeling through prior fractures and dislocations regions.

Chronic CN deformities are typically corrected with some form of osteotomy and arthrodesis procedures. Often, the deformities involved have a distorted osseous contour and integrity when compared with normal bony structures. Bone resection through the apex of the deformity that is combined with an arthrodesis procedure is typically performed to create a plantigrade foot and to ultimately achieve a better alignment of the foot to the leg. At times for severe midfoot deformities, wide resection through the tarsal bones with resection of remaining cartilage and shortening of the foot can provide laxity of the soft tissues to achieve resolution of ulcers that are present. In addition, tarsal bones may have to be resected in the presence of avascular necrosis, and the osseous contour is not amenable to an anatomic arthrodesis procedure.

Peritalar deformities that involve the ankle and hindfoot can be managed with talectomy and tibiocalcaneal arthrodesis, tibiotalocalcaneal arthrodesis, and/or pantalar arthrodesis if the talus is deemed salvageable. Often, the talus is avascular from the CN process, and talectomy with tibiocalcaneal arthrodesis is required (**Fig. 3**). Surgical techniques in these cases involve bone and joint resection with contouring of the bony segments to achieve an acceptable alignment. Autogenous and/or allogenic bone grafting along with orthobiologics can be used to enhance bone healing. Regardless of the fixation chosen to achieve stability, emphasis on surgical incision placement, bone resection, removal of necrotic bone, and meticulous joint preparation cannot be overemphasized.

The role of tendon balancing procedures in select case scenarios must also be considered. Equinus contracture is common among midfoot rocker-bottom deformities, and commonly a percutaneous tendo-Achilles lengthening or tenotomy versus gastrocnemius recession is performed. One must also consider the possibility of over-lengthening and creation of a calcaneal gait that may lead to heel ulceration. For this reason, the role for equinus correction is debatable and should be performed on a case-by-case basis. Certain clinical scenarios warrant an adjunctive tenotomy to other major foot tendons in addition to the osseous reconstruction for balancing of the deforming forces. For example, patients with ulcerations to the plantar lateral midfoot region that have had prior fifth metatarsal base region infection and resection of osseous/soft tissue structures that resulted in loss of the peroneal brevis tendon attachment and CN deformity are difficult to manage. Varus deformity progresses in this patient population as a result of the pull of the posterior tibial tendon. In these cases, it is beneficial to perform a posterior tibial tendon tenotomy in addition to the osseous correction to prevent recurrent varus deformity. In addition, the tibialis anterior tendon has been reported to have ruptured with a chronic CN deformity resulting

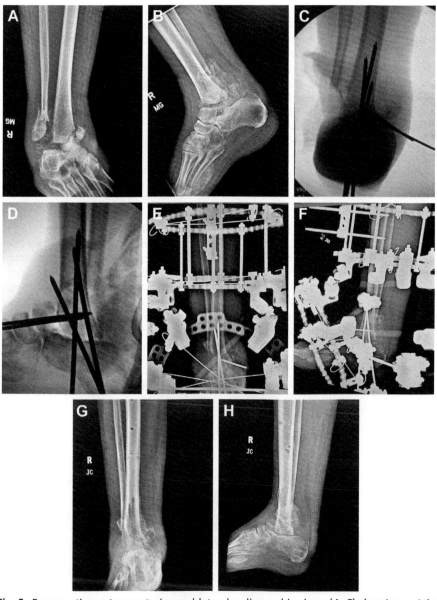

Fig. 3. Preoperative anteroposterior and lateral radiographic views (*A, B*) showing a right ankle and hindfoot CN with a distal tibia/fibula and talus fractures. Patient underwent a talectomy with tibiocalcaneal arthrodesis (*C, D*) and application of a multiplanar circular external fixation (*E, F*). Final radiographic views at 6 months postoperatively demonstrating a stable and well-aligned tibiocalcaneal pseudoarthrosis (*G, H*). Functional ambulation permitted with high-top custom-made diabetic shoes with inlays and double upright brace to the right lower extremity.

in a midfoot deformity and foot drop.[10] An extensor hallucis longus tendon transfer in addition to a midfoot reconstruction was performed in this unique clinical scenario.

Internal and external fixation techniques have been described during CN reconstruction. Typically, standard internal fixation techniques, such as lag screws (for interfragmentary compression) with or without standard plate fixation, are often not sufficient to stabilize CN-related fractures or dislocations. Bridge plating is a useful technique because it extends past the zone of injury both proximally and distally using less-affected bone to achieve better screw fixation. Plantar plating has been described to provide superior strength by applying the plate to the tension side of the bone. Medial plating for midfoot deformities has been described to address severe transverse plane CN deformities and to provide stability to multiple midfoot joints. Locking plates can be used, combining locking and nonlocking in osteopenic bone that will create a more rigid construct. Blade plating is another option for hindfoot/ankle procedures that provides a fixed angle construct to increase stability of the arthrodesis site (**Fig. 4**).

With any type of plating system, it requires an adequate soft tissue envelope. Intramedullary metatarsal screws or intramedullary foot nails allow for a more limited open approach for the fixation where the hardware is intraosseous. Although beaming screws and nails in the foot have been reported in the literature, the authors of this article do not advocate their use because they have encountered revisional surgeries with beaming screws in place that posed problems for removal and revisional surgery. Intramedullary nail for hindfoot/ankle arthrodesis can be used to achieve rigid hindfoot/ankle stabilization, which is preferred with the authors of this article when good bone stock is present, and the patient is free of infection.

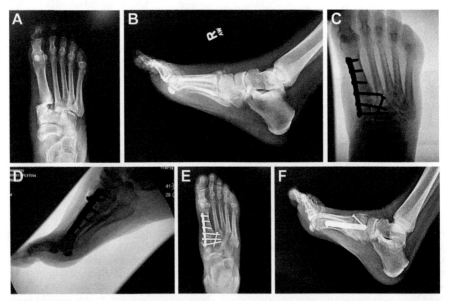

Fig. 4. Preoperative anteroposterior and lateral radiographic views (*A, B*) of an acute/subacute right midfoot CN with fracture, dislocation, and instability. Treatment options were discussed with the patient, and surgical intervention was performed with an open reduction internal fixation and primary Lisfranc joint arthrodesis (*C, D*). Final radiographic views demonstrate successful arthrodesis (*E, F*). Patient was ambulating in diabetic shoes with custom-made inlays.

External fixation for CN has shown good results in patients with severe bone loss, osteopenic bone, osteomyelitis, peripheral vascular disease, previous failed internal fixation, and poor soft tissue envelope. Circular external fixation allows one to span the deformity away from the zone of injury and provides stability and compression at the arthrodesis site along with stabilization of the foot to the leg, which will maintain correction over a period of time. Circular external fixators provide a rigid, stable construct through the use of transosseous wires and half-pins. They are a versatile tool to use with these cases, as one is able to correct deformities while simultaneously providing stability to the lower extremity along with compression to an arthrodesis when needed. Various external fixation constructs can be designed to midfoot, rearfoot, and/or ankle CN deformities.

Static circular external fixators can be used for additional stability of the lower extremity, for surgical offloading of the soft tissues, to provide access to an ulcer to perform wound care, to augment the underlying fixation, and to avoid splinting/casting. They are typically assembled with a combination of a tibial block (1 or 2 tibial rings) and a foot plate or ring.[12–14] These circular external fixators can be modified to each patient to aid in further stability and offloading. Hybrid constructs have been described that incorporate circular rings with a bar to clap apparatus. Dynamic circular external fixators have also been described that require gradual deformity correction to obtain joint realignment. Detailed surgical planning and creative foresight are imperative in choosing the best construct for each individual patient that sometimes may combine internal and external fixation systems.

Evolving techniques have focused on increasing stability of fixation primarily by extending hardware proximally and distally into areas where the bone is not fragmented by the neuropathic process. Superconstructs may be used to describe this technique to extend the arthrodesis site to include adjacent joins to prevent nonunion and further deformity. Superconstructs are defined by 4 characteristics or principles in the literature: arthrodesis is extended beyond the zone of injury to include joints that are not affected to improve fixation; bone resection performed to shorten the extremity to allow for adequate reduction of deformity without undue tension on the soft tissue envelope; the strongest device is used that can be tolerated by the soft tissue envelope; and devices are applied in a position that maximizes mechanical function.[15–19] Disadvantages of this technique, though, are larger surgical exposures and increased operating time.

The role of major amputation for the management of CN may be indicated with sepsis, active infection to the extremity, severe peripheral arterial disease, failed prior surgeries, severe bone loss, patient preference, and poor ambulatory potential.[20]

POSTOPERATIVE CARE

Postoperative care is critical to minimize complications and to have successful outcomes. Patient compliance is essential, as patients need to be thoroughly educated on their requirements and responsibilities. Non-weight-bearing restrictions can vary from 2 to 5 months on average for this condition. No standard of care exists for deep venous thrombosis prophylaxis and is often determined based on the patient's risk factors. In certain instances, patients are placed on low-molecular-weight heparin initially and then transitioned to an aspirin twice a day until they are ambulatory into shoe gear, unless they need to resume other anticoagulation medications based on the medical team recommendations.

Pin site care varies in patients with external fixation. The authors' preference is to wrap the external fixator in sterile dressings to prevent pin site irritation and infection.

The pins are commonly inspected every 2 weeks until incision/wound healing and then every 4 weeks until osseous healing and plan for removal of the external fixator. These devices are typically removed in the operating room, and any additional wound issues if present can be addressed at that time if needed. After the external fixator is removed, casts and further immobilization are carried out until patients are transitioned into appropriate shoe gear and/or bracing.

SUMMARY

CN is a potentially limb-threatening condition. The goal of treatment is to provide a stable plantigrade foot that allows for functional ambulation and no ulceration. CN requires a clear understanding of the pathophysiology of the disease process as it progress from acute to chronic stages. When surgery is indicated, the choice of fixation, whether internal, external, or a combination of the two, should be applied to provide osseous stability that also accounts for anticipated problems and soft tissue concerns commonly seen in the management of this condition.

Despite the advances of fixation constructs, emphasis is still placed on basic surgical principles to achieve deformity correction through precise osteotomies and meticulous joint preparation for joint arthrodesis. Surgery for CN is not for all patients, and some patients may simply prefer amputation as opposed to the lengthy recovery involved with attempted limb salvage procedures. Thorough education and discussion with the patient on limb salvage options and amputation allow the patient to make an informed decision on their care. Also, complications can present among the surgical management of these patients, and achieving limb salvage is often dependent on the management of these complications.

REFERENCES

1. Elbert D, Langan T, Burns P. Surgical treatment and management of chronic dislocated subtalar joint. J Foot Ankle Surg 2020;59:379–84.
2. Papa J, Myerson M, Girard P. Salvage, with arthrodesis, in intractable diabetic neuropathic arthropathy of the foot and ankle. J Bone Joint Surg 1993;75(7):1056–66.
3. Jolly GP, Zgonis T, Polyzois V. External fixation in the management of Charcot neuroarthropathy. Clin Podiatr Med Surg 2003;20(4):741–56.
4. Pakarinen TK, Laine HJ, Honkonen SE, et al. Charcot arthropathy of the diabetic foot. Current concepts and review of 36 cases. Scand J Surg 2002;91:195–201.
5. Lee L, Blume PA, Sumpio B. Charcot joint disease in diabetes mellitus. Ann Vasc Surg 2003;17(5):571–80.
6. Yu GV, Hudson JR. Evaluation and treatment of stage 0 Charcot's neuroarthropathy of the foot and ankle. J Am Podiatr Med Assoc 2002;92(4):210–20.
7. Trepman E, Nihal A, Pinzur MS. Current topics review: Charcot neuroarthropathy of the foot and ankle. Foot Ankle Int 2005;26(1):46–63.
8. Simon SR, Tejwani SG, Wilson DL, et al. Arthrodesis as an early alternative to nonoperative management of Charcot arthropathy of the diabetic foot. J Bone Joint Surg 2000;82-A(7):939–50.
9. Marmolejo VS, Arnold J, Ponticello J, et al. Charcot foot: clinical clues, diagnostic strategies, and treatment principles. Am Fam Physician 2018;97(9):594–9.
10. Stapleton JJ. Simultaneous surgical repair of a tibialis anterior tendon rupture and diabetic Charcot neuroarthropathy of the midfoot, a case report. Clin Podiatric Med Surg 2013;30(4):599–604.

11. Ahmadi ME, Morrison WB, Carrino JA, et al. Neuropathic arthropathy of the foot with and without superimposed osteomyelitis: MR imaging characteristics. Radiology 2006;238(2):622–31.
12. Lowenberg DW, Sadeghi C, Brooks D, et al. Use of circular external fixation to maintain foot position during free tissue transfer to the foot and ankle. Microsurgery 2008;28(8):623–7.
13. Zgonis T, Roukis TS, Stapleton JJ, et al. Combined lateral column arthrodesis, medial plantar artery flap, and circular external fixation for Charcot midfoot collapse with chronic plantar ulceration. Adv Skin Wound Care 2008;21(11): 521–5.
14. Ergen FB, Sanverdi SE, Oznur A. Charcot foot in diabetes and an update on imaging. Diabetes Foot & Ankle 2013;4:21884.
15. Sammarco VJ. Supercontructs in the treatment of Charcot foot deformity; plantar plating, locked plating, and axial screw fixation. Foot Ankle Clin 2009;14(3): 393–407.
16. Hegewald KE, Wilder ML, Chappell TM, et al. Combined internal and external fixation for diabetic Charcot reconstruction: a retrospective case series. J Foot Ankle Surg 2016;55(3):619–27.
17. Burns PR, Wukich DK. Surgical reconstruction of the Charcot rearfoot and ankle. Clin Podiatric Med Surg 2008;25:95–120.
18. Stapleton JJ, Zgonis T. Surgical reconstruction of the diabetic Charcot foot: internal, external or combined fixation? Clin Podiatric Med Surg 2012;29:425–33.
19. Pinzur MS, Shields N, Trepman E, et al. Current practice patterns in the treatment of Charcot foot. Foot Ankle Int 2000;21:916–20.
20. Ramanujam C, Facaros Z, Zgonis T. External fixation for surgical off-loading of diabetic soft tissue reconstruction. Clin Podiatric Med Surg 2011;28:211–6.

Soft Tissue and Osseous Substitutes for the Diabetic Foot

Steven L. Stuto, DPM, Crystal L. Ramanujam, DPM, MSc*,
Thomas Zgonis, DPM

KEYWORDS

• Orthobiologics • Diabetic foot • Wound • Bone • Allograft • Neuropathy

KEY POINTS

• Soft tissue and osseous substitutes provide adjunctive options for surgical reconstruction of diabetic foot and ankle wounds.
• Medical optimization and acute infection should be addressed before considering the use of soft tissue and/or osseous substitutes.
• With careful patient selection, advanced soft tissue and osseous orthobiologics can be used in combination with other reconstructive procedures to provide wound closure and restore structure and function of the diabetic foot.

Diabetic foot infections and osteomyelitis are a challenge because initial infection control with aggressive surgical debridement can lead to soft tissue compromise and osseous deficits. The literature reports that approximately 25% of diabetic patients will develop a wound in their lifetime due to peripheral neuropathy, vascular disease, or combination of both, and more than half of these patients become infected.[1–5] Complete eradication of all nonviable soft tissue and bone without a major concern of limb length discrepancy or soft tissue compromise is the initial step to treat a diabetic foot infection. Following this, surgeons are faced with an opportune situation: choose between resecting more to make surgical wound closure easier or consider delayed closure with a soft tissue or bone substitute and reconstructive techniques to help heal the large deficit and increasing the patient's potential for rehabilitation and mobility.

One of the most significant factors for a successful soft tissue or osseous healing in a diabetic patient with multiple medical comorbidities is a healthy wound bed and joint preparation before the use of any soft tissue or osseous substitute. Multiple staged surgical debridements and wound bed preparations might be necessary before the

Division of Podiatric Medicine and Surgery, Department of Orthopaedics, University of Texas Health San Antonio, 7703 Floyd Curl Drive, MC 7776, San Antonio, TX 78229, USA
* Corresponding author.
E-mail address: Ramanujam@uthscsa.edu

Clin Podiatr Med Surg 39 (2022) 343–350
https://doi.org/10.1016/j.cpm.2021.11.006
0891-8422/22/© 2021 Elsevier Inc. All rights reserved.

definitive reconstructive procedure. Additional prerequisites to the final reconstruction include the following: addressing the underlying vascular insufficiency, uncontrolled hyperglycemia, nutritional deficiency, and overall medical status of the patient. Equally important is correcting the underlying lower extremity deformity, osseous prominence, equinus contracture, and instability at the time of index surgery that is free of any soft tissue or osseous infection.

Medical optimization and consultation with specialties such as cardiology, endocrinology, nephrology, vascular surgery, and infectious disease when deemed necessary will benefit the patient to a healthy recovery and understanding of the entire health care team effort to prevent complications such as a major lower extremity amputation. For example, in cases that are not urgent/emergent and require surgical intervention, the definitive procedure may be delayed until the patient is medically optimized with recommendations from health care providers who are actively involved in the patient's care. Often, an echocardiography, coronary or lower extremity angiography, change in the patient's insulin regimen or anticoagulation therapy, and coordination with patient's hemodialysis schedule might be performed before the patient's reconstruction. It is also equally important that the patient and patient's family members are well-educated with the patient's condition and treatment methods throughout the preoperative process and preparation for surgery, anesthesia, and strict postoperative protocol with most likely prolonged non-weight-bearing status, rehabilitation, and antibiotic therapy.

In contrast, diabetic patients who present with urgent/emergent conditions such as necrotizing fasciitis and severe foot and ankle infections with purulence, abscess, osteomyelitis, and sepsis, an expedited surgical intervention may be required with the input of medical and/or anesthesiology services. Once the patient is hemodynamically stable after the initial urgent/emergent intervention, staged procedures may be performed during the same hospitalization with the medical optimization provided by the necessary services. In certain cases, definitive procedures may be delayed after the patient's hospital discharge when the surgical wounds are prepared with maximum blood supply and free of infection (**Fig. 1**).

SOFT TISSUE SUBSTITUTES

Soft tissue substitutes have augmented the treatment of diabetic foot and ankle wounds by giving the option to either prevent or delay a more invasive surgical intervention for closure. Martinson and Martinson[3] reported that diabetic foot wounds failed to heal 24% to 60% of the time, and adjunctive treatment with skin grafts and skin substitutes could increase the healing rate of diabetic foot ulcerations. Sabolinski and Capotorto[5] reported that 70% of diabetic foot ulcerations do not respond to standard care and need a biologic to jump-start the healing process. Clerici and colleagues[6] reported that 87% of all wounds healed with their protocol of applying a dermal substitute graft at the second stage and later performing a split-thickness skin graft at 21 days. In addition, Clerici and colleagues[6] reported the use of dermal substitutes for exposed healthy tendon and bone following surgical debridement as a treatment in cases of foot infection instead of a more proximal amputation to preserve length and function.[6]

Skin substitutes that can be used to facilitate wound healing and several engineered substitutes are commercially available. Apligraf (Graftskin; Organogenesis, Inc, Canton, MA, USA) is a composite allograft comprising bovine type 1 collagen gel and living neonatal fibroblasts as the dermal component, with an epidermal layer composed of neonatal keratinocytes.[1] These allografts can be applied on uninfected partial-thickness or full-thickness diabetic foot wounds, but multiple applications of

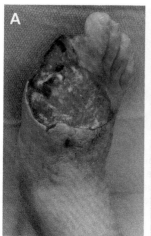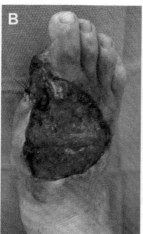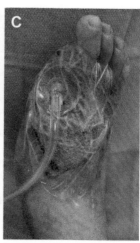

Fig. 1. Intraoperative picture (*A*) of a diabetic patient who underwent an urgent/emergent right foot hallux amputation and excisional debridement that was followed by a revisional excisional debridement, partial resection of the first metatarsal (*B*), and application of a negative pressure wound therapy (*C*) during the same hospital stay. Definitive wound closure of a large soft tissue defect can be performed after the patient's hospital discharge, which may entail the use of allogenic or autogenous split-thickness skin grafting procedures.

Apligraf may be needed to achieve complete healing.[7] Dermagraft (Advanced Bio-Healing, Inc, La Jolla, CA, USA) is one such allograft made from neonatal fibroblasts seeded onto a resorbable polyglactin polymer scaffold and is indicated for the treatment of chronic diabetic foot wounds without exposed bone, tendon, capsule, or muscle and typically requires multiple applications.[8] EpiFix (MiMedx, Kennesaw, GA, USA) is a dehydrated form of human amniotic membrane that has preserved the properties of the natural membrane yet having a stable shelf life of 5 years at room temperature.[9] Several commercially available amniotic membrane-derived grafts available are composed of structural collagen, extracellular matrix, biologically active cells, and regenerative molecules, and are indicated for neuropathic diabetic foot ulcerations.

Synthetic bilayer substitutes are acellular products that serve as dermal matrices that promote ingrowth of host tissues to repair defects. Integra bilayer matrix wound dressing (Integra LifeSciences Corp, Plainsboro, NJ, USA) is composed of an outer silicone sheet with an underlying bovine collagen and glycosaminoglycan matrix.[1] These grafts are indicated for noninfected deep diabetic wounds, such as those after partial foot amputation, and surgical wounds at flap donor sites that are not amenable to autogenous skin grafting (**Figs. 2** and **3**). Ramanujam and colleagues[2] reported the use of negative pressure wound therapy and then application of acellular dermal replacement graft to achieve primary closure in extensive diabetic foot wounds. Santema and colleagues[4] concluded that a multidisciplinary approach is needed when applying skin substitutes. GRAFTJACKET (Wright Medical Technology, Inc, LifeCell Corporation for Kinetic Concepts Inc, Arlington, TN, USA) is another acellular dermal allograft that has been processed to remove living cells, preserving an intact matrix that supports repopulation and revascularization by the recipient tissue, and is indicated for use in lower extremity wounds in patients with diabetes.[1] Overall, the use of skin substitutes has been associated with fewer dressing changes, shorter hospital stays, shorter offloading periods, and a protection barrier against wound infection.

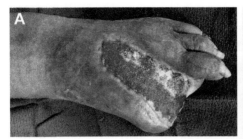
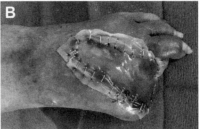

Fig. 2. Intraoperative picture (*A*) of a diabetic patient with a history of a left foot partial amputation that was managed with negative pressure wound therapy and local wound care that underwent hydrosurgical wound bed preparation and application of a bilayer matrix wound dressing (*B*). Note the adequate granulation tissue and minimal fibrotic tissue of the chronically open wound free of infection (*A*) and before use of a soft tissue substitute (*B*).

Soft tissue substitutes can be used in combination with other surgical procedures for diabetic foot and ankle wounds such as to cover donor sites from flap reconstruction (**Fig. 4**).

Osseous Substitutes

Increased rates of nonunion have been reported for diabetic patients undergoing any type of foot and/or ankle fusion.[10] Although autogenous bone graft remains the gold standard, it may have limited availability and can be associated with increased morbidity and extended surgical times.[7] Osteoconductive agents serve as a scaffold matrix for cells to infiltrate and allow growth across the material, and osteoinductive agents are growth factors that stimulate nondifferentiated mesenchymal cells to differentiate into osteoblasts and other bone- or cartilage-forming cells.[10] Osteobiologic agents that have been useful for diabetic foot and ankle surgery include structural allografts, demineralized bone matrix (DBM), and bone morphogenetic proteins (BMPs).

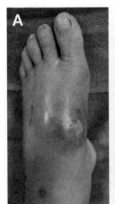
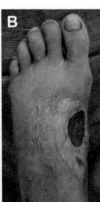
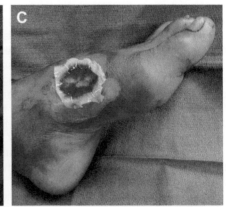

Fig. 3. Intraoperative picture (*A*) of a diabetic patient who underwent an urgent/emergent excisional debridement that was followed by a revisional excisional debridement (*B*) and application of a bilayer matrix wound dressing (*C*) during the same hospital stay. Note the healthy tissue at the recipient wound bed that is small in size and before use of a soft tissue substitute (*C*).

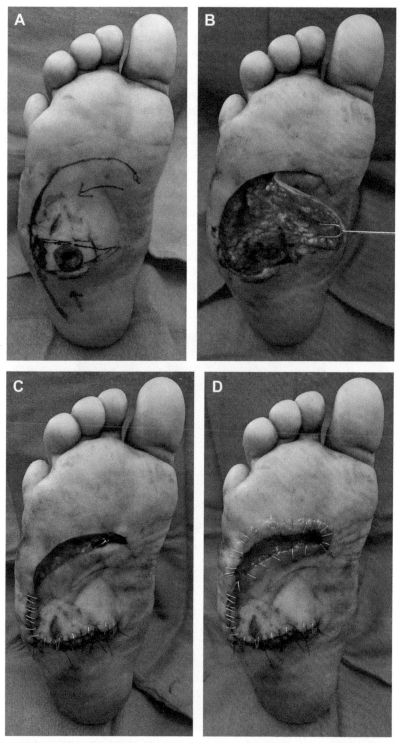

Fig. 4. Intraoperative picture (*A*) of a diabetic patient with Charcot neuroarthropathy and a chronic nonhealing wound who underwent a reverse flow fasciocutaneous flap based on the medial plantar artery (*B, C*). Note the use of a bilayer matrix wound dressing to cover the donor site of the flap closure (*D*).

DBM and BMPs can be easily combined with autologous or allogenic bone graft material for use in corrective arthrodesis and/or the treatment of nonunions.[11] Available bone allograft types include cancellous or cortical bone, cadaveric bone (typically fresh-frozen or freeze-dried), and demineralized and synthetic bone grafts. Bone graft substitutes contribute an advantage in diabetic foot and ankle reconstruction because they have an unlimited amount of product to augment large defects and enhance bone healing.[11] (**Fig. 5**).

Most of the research on bone graft substitutes for diabetic foot and ankle surgery is centered around inorganic bioceramics, calcium phosphate, calcium sulfate, and hydroxyapatite (HA). In the diabetic Charcot neuroarthropathy of the foot and ankle in the presence or absence of osteomyelitis, bone loss is a significant barrier to care; therefore, calcium phosphate, calcium sulfate, and HA coupled with antibiotic powder can be used to fill the bone void in addition to treating osteomyelitis. HA is the most osteoconductive of all calcium phosphates and is commonly combined with calcium sulfate to increase the resorption rate. Nilsson and colleagues[12] reported the use of 5 mL HA/calcium sulfate paste for metatarsal delayed union with success of bone callus formation. The investigators also reported forefoot osteomyelitis and the use of HA/calcium sulfate impregnated with vancomycin with no recurrence of osteomyelitis at 6 months

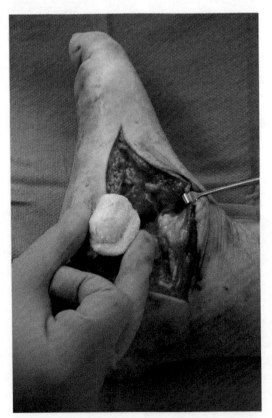

Fig. 5. Intraoperative picture of a diabetic patient with Charcot neuroarthropathy preparing a medial column arthrodesis with resection of the cartilaginous surfaces and application of allogenic bone grafting before circular external fixation utilization.

postoperatively.[12] Hollawell[13] reported a 100% fusion rate in 20 patients using autograft alternative Osteocel Plus (NuVasive, Inc, San Diego, CA, USA), which is an allogenic cellular bone matrix for hindfoot and ankle fusions; however, not all the subjects had diabetes mellitus.

For reconstructive cases of the diabetic Charcot foot and ankle, allogenic bone grafting becomes ideal in the presence of large osseous defects encountered by procedures such as a talectomy performed to address a hindfoot/ankle deformity with a tibiocalcaneal arthrodesis. When concomitant osteomyelitis is present, all the infected and nonviable bone needs to be resected if feasible and also be managed with systemic antibiotic therapy and/or local antibiotic delivery when indicated. The resected joints with osteomyelitis can be initially augmented with the use of cemented nonbiodegradable antibiotic beads or spacers for local antibiotic delivery and soft tissue and osseous stabilization. Adjunctive therapies such as negative pressure wound therapy and/or external fixation for surgical offloading might be indicated in certain clinical case scenarios with severe instability and large soft tissue and osseous defects. After eradication of the infected underlying osseous structures, allogenic bone grafting can be used for the definitive arthrodesis procedure with the use of external fixation or selective internal fixation when deemed necessary.

SUMMARY

Soft tissue and osseous substitutes have drastically increased options for diabetic foot and ankle surgery because they help to incorporate enhanced healing potential and promote safety as alternatives to more invasive procedures or may also be used in combination with other reconstructive techniques. The use of these products in diabetic limb salvage is best carried out with careful patient selection in a multidisciplinary approach consisting of initial medical optimization with glycemic control, surgical debridement and antibiotic therapy to resolve infection, adequate arterial perfusion, effective offloading, and continuous patient education.

REFERENCES

1. Ramanujam CL, Zgonis T. An overview of autologous skin grafts and advanced biologics for the diabetic foot. Clin Podiatr Med Surg 2012;29(3):435–41.
2. Ramanujam CL, Capobianco CM, Zgonis T. Using a bilayer matrix wound dressing for closure of complicated diabetic foot wounds. J Wound Care 2010; 19(2):56–60.
3. Martinson M, Martinson N. A comparative analysis of skin substitutes used in the management of diabetic foot ulcers. J Wound Care 2016;25(Suppl10):S8–17.
4. Santema TB, Poyck PP, Ubbink DT. Systematic review and meta-analysis of skin substitutes in the treatment of diabetic foot ulcers: highlights of a cochrane systematic review. Wound Repair Regen 2016;24(4):737–44.
5. Sabolinski ML, Capotorto JV. Comparative effectiveness of a human fibroblast-derived dermal substitute and a viable cryopreserved placental membrane for the treatment of diabetic foot ulcers. J Comp Eff Res 2019;8(14):1229–38.
6. Clerici G, Caminiti M, Curci V, et al. The use of a dermal substitute to preserve maximal foot length in diabetic foot wounds with tendon and bone exposure following urgent surgical debridement for acute infection. Int Wound J 2010; 7(3):176–83.
7. Veves A, Falanga V, Armstrong DG, et al. Apligraf Diabetic Foot Ulcer Study. Graftskin, a human skin equivalent, is effective in the management of noninfected

neuropathic diabetic foot ulcers: a prospective randomized multicenter clinical trial. Diabetes Care 2001;24(2):290–5.

8. Marston WA, Hanft J, Norwood P, et al. Dermagraft Diabetic Foot Ulcer Study Group. The efficacy and safety of Dermagraft in improving the healing of chronic diabetic foot ulcers: results of a prospective randomized trial. Diabetes Care 2003;26(6):1701–5.

9. Zelen CM, Serena TE, Denoziere G, et al. A prospective randomised comparative parallel study of amniotic membrane wound graft in the management of diabetic foot ulcers. Int Wound J 2013;10(5):502–7.

10. Rabinovich RV, Haleem AM, Rozbruch SR. Complex ankle arthrodesis: review of the literature. World J Orthop 2015;6(8):602–13.

11. Ramanujam CL, Facaros Z, Zgonis T. An overview of bone grafting techniques for the diabetic Charcot foot and ankle. Clin Podiatr Med Surg 2012;29(4):589–95.

12. Nilsson M, Zheng MH, Tägil M. The composite of hydroxyapatite and calcium sulphate: a review of preclinical evaluation and clinical applications. Expert Rev Med Devices 2013;10(5):675–84.

13. Hollawell SM. Allograft cellular bone matrix as an alternative to autograft in hindfoot and ankle fusion procedures. J Foot Ankle Surg 2012;51(2):222–5.

External Fixation for Surgical Offloading of the Diabetic Foot

Hani M. Badahdah, DPM, MD, MS[a,b,]*, Thomas Zgonis, DPM[c]

KEYWORDS

- Diabetic foot • Surgical offloading • External fixation • Ulcer • Flaps

KEY POINTS

- Surgical offloading of the foot and ankle with external fixation may be considered in carefully selected diabetic patients who have failed to heal through conservative methods.
- External fixation for the diabetic foot has been reported for several clinical scenarios in addition to isolated surgical offloading including management of osteomyelitis and bone defects, complex arthrodesis, and deformity correction such as Charcot neuroarthropathy.
- A multidisciplinary team approach should be used for high-risk diabetic patients being considered for surgical reconstruction, especially in the use of circular external fixation to reduce the risk of complications.

Diabetic foot ulcerations and infections are a frequent source of morbidity including a leading cause of hospital admission and may lead to lower extremity amputation. Peripheral neuropathy and plantar pressure alteration are responsible for most diabetic foot ulcerations. If the ulceration is caused by an osseous deformity and/or biomechanical abnormalities, nonsurgical treatment options may include traditional offloading techniques such as total contact casting, below-the-knee casting or splints, stabilizing walkers/shoes, whereas surgical options may include corrective procedures underlying any osseous/soft tissue abnormalities and use of surgical offloading.[1,2] Complex diabetic foot wounds with infection, vascular compromise, and unstable osseous deformity may require staged surgical procedures and a longer period of wound healing to salvage the lower extremity.[1]

Diabetic limb salvage with surgical reconstruction of complex diabetic foot wounds is best approached with a multidisciplinary team effort including but not limited to

[a] Dr.Edrees Specialized Medical Center, Prince Sultan Road, Jeddah 23423, Saudi Arabia; [b] Diabetes and Endocrinology Center, King Fahd Specialist Hospital, King Abdullah Road, Buraydah 52366, Saudi Arabia; [c] Reconstructive Foot and Ankle Surgery Fellowship, Division of Podiatric Medicine and Surgery, Department of Orthopaedics, University of Texas Health San Antonio, 7703 Floyd Curl Drive, MC 7776, San Antonio, TX 78229, USA
* Corresponding author. Diabetes and Endocrinology Center, King Fahd Specialist Hospital, King Abdullah Road, Buraydah 52366, Saudi Arabia
E-mail address: badahdahdpm@gmail.com

Clin Podiatr Med Surg 39 (2022) 351–356
https://doi.org/10.1016/j.cpm.2021.11.007
0891-8422/22/© 2021 Elsevier Inc. All rights reserved.

vascular interventionists to establish adequate blood flow for wound healing, reconstructive foot and ankle surgeons to stabilize osseous deformities through external fixation, infectious disease specialists to address any residual infection, medicine, endocrinology, nephrology, and cardiology to manage any pre-existed medical comorbidities.[1,3] Although surgical intervention may be considered high risk in this patient population, the reported outcomes have been acceptable and predictable when patients are carefully selected along with surgical experience and specializing training in the application of external fixation. In the absence of effective surgical offloading after osseous, soft-tissue, and/or flap reconstruction, the wound healing process can be delayed and interrupted with more complications.

Major lower extremity amputation may be considered as a faster solution for complicated wounds with underlying infections that may enable some patients to ambulate in a short period with an expedited recovery. However, the risks of a major amputation in a diabetic patient with multiple comorbidities including cardiac, renal, and peripheral vascular disease cannot be overlooked as it is associated with increased health care costs, decreased life expectancy, and increased risk of complications and contralateral limb amputation.[1,2]

SURGICAL CONSIDERATIONS

Diabetic patients undergoing surgical reconstruction may require multiple procedures and are often at high risk for surgery and anesthesia because of their multiple medical comorbidities; therefore, a multidisciplinary team is required to optimize and manage the comorbidities before any surgical intervention.[4] Necessary consultations and recommendations from the medical and anesthesiology teams based on the patient's surgical procedure and anesthesia demands are vital to the patient's successful recovery.

A detailed medical and surgical history should be obtained with careful physical examination of the patient's wound characteristics, with vascular, neurologic, and orthopedic assessments. Any previous surgeries, history of open wounds, retained hardware, medical allergies, problems with anesthesia, blood transfusions, history of deep vein thrombosis, pulmonary embolism, vascular/cardiac interventions, or hemodialysis are important factors to consider before proceeding with the proposed surgical procedure. Laboratory investigations and medical imaging testing should be obtained and interpreted carefully. Thorough discussions with the patient about the entire process of medical optimization, surgical reconstruction, external fixation application, extended period of non–weight-bearing status, rehabilitation, social/family support, compliance, expectations, and goals of surgery may help the patient understand the proposed plan in a more efficient way while reducing the risk of postoperative complications.

There are multiple external fixation configurations for surgical offloading and the most common one used for diabetic limb salvage procedures includes a multiplanar circular external fixation that allows for a simultaneous osseous deformity and soft tissue correction. The duration of circular external fixation utilization for surgical offloading depends on the associated simultaneous procedural selection and can range from 8 to 12 weeks. After removal of the external fixation device, the patient can be placed in a below-the-knee cast or posterior splint for immobilization and then gradually advance to ambulation with a stabilizing walker. Long-term, custom-made shoes, orthotics, and bracing should be prescribed to stabilize and maintain correction of the lower extremity while preventing ulceration recurrence.

CASE REPORT

A 55-year-old male patient presented with a history of a recalcitrant neuropathic non-healing wound on the plantar lateral aspect of the right foot for 3 years (**Fig. 1**A). An

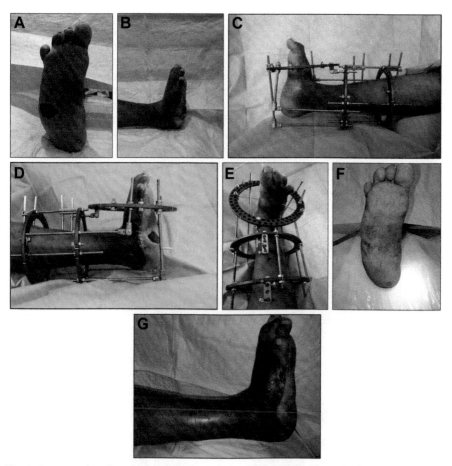

Fig. 1. Preoperative picture of a diabetic patient with a history of a right foot partial amputation for osteomyelitis with chronic plantar ulceration (*A*) and equinocavovarus deformity (*B*). Intraoperative pictures (*C–E*) of the patient who underwent excisional debridement with resection of cuboid bone, application of antibiotic-impregnated cemented beads, percutaneous tendo-Achilles lengthening, posterior tibial tenotomy, and application of a circular external fixation for surgical offloading. Postoperative pictures of the patient following removal of the circular external fixation with complete healing of the wound (*F*) and correction of the deformity (*G*).

equinocavovarus deformity had resulted after fourth and fifth metatarsal complete resection for osteomyelitis (**Fig. 1B**). His past medical history consisted of poorly controlled type 2 diabetes mellitus and hypertension. Past conservative treatments including total contact casting, stabilizing walker, offloading shoes, wound care, and long-term antibiotics had failed to heal the open wound and he was also offered a major amputation as a treatment option.

At initial presentation, a chronic nonhealing wound on the plantar lateral aspect of the right foot with purulence drainage and probing deep to the cuboid bone level was noted. His vascular status was intact with palpable dorsalis pedis and posterior tibial arteries. Based on the patient's medical status, laboratory results, radiologic findings, and wound characteristics, surgical intervention was recommended for limb salvage. The surgical plan included a surgical debridement, resection of cuboid bone due to osteomyelitis, application of antibiotic-impregnated cemented beads, percutaneous tendo-Achilles lengthening, posterior tibial tenotomy, and application of multiplane circular external fixation (**Fig.** 1C–E). The patient elected to proceed with surgery and the procedures were performed under spinal anesthesia with utilization of a thigh tourniquet. The circular external fixator was maintained for 8 weeks until complete wound healing and then removed (**Fig.** 1F, G). Serial postoperative casting was performed for 1 month and then the patient was allowed to bear weight gradually using a stabilizing walker. Eventually, the patient was placed in an extra-depth custom-made high-top diabetic shoe at approximately 4 months from the index surgery and without reulceration at his final follow-up visit.

DISCUSSION

Management of chronic diabetic foot ulcerations can be a challenge and often requires a multidisciplinary approach to optimize wound healing by addressing comorbidities, improving arterial perfusion, and eliminating infection. Initially, conservative

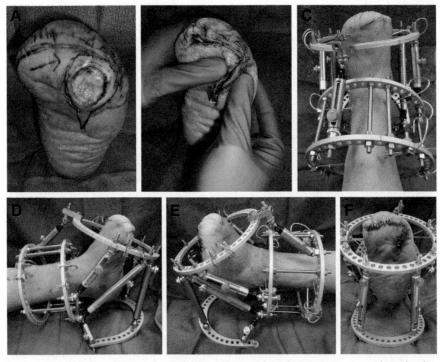

Fig. 2. Intraoperative picture of a diabetic patient with a chronic open wound nonhealing at the transmetatarsal amputation (A) after multiple failed conservative treatments of casting/splinting, local wound care, and antibiotic therapy. The patient underwent a single local random rotational flap closure (B) with an application of a circular external fixation device for surgical offloading (C–F). Note that medial and lateral struts (D, E) placement that allow for correction of any associated varus/valgus and equinus deformity with simultaneous osseous/soft-tissue procedures and the struts that are used for surgical offloading (F) elevating the heel from any contact surfaces by preventing a weight-bearing status and allowing for direct visualization of the flap and access to local wound care if needed.

offloading is used to protect lower extremity wounds against direct and indirect pressures. However, traditional offloading may be inadequate in cases of complicated wounds with osseous deformity, compromised soft tissue, persistent infection, and excessive edema. If conservative offloading fails, external fixation may be a viable option in the carefully selected patient.[3,4] The use of external fixation is an effective technique that can help patients who have difficulty with other offloading methods such as casting or splinting (**Fig. 2**). External fixation allows complete offloading of the lower extremity and discourages weight-bearing.[5] This provides an optimal environment for wound healing simultaneously through offloading, immobilizing joints, and stabilizing osseous deformity. Application of external fixation in exposed and unstable joints

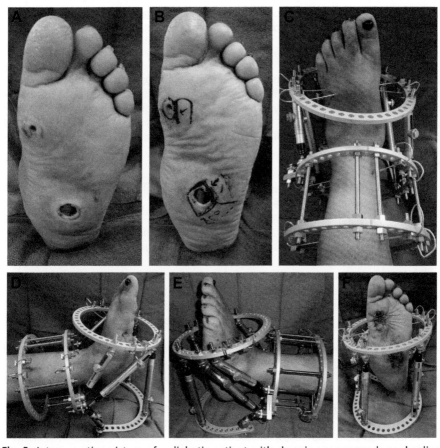

Fig. 3. Intraoperative picture of a diabetic patient with chronic open wounds nonhealing and Charcot neuroarthropathy (*A*) after multiple failed conservative treatments of casting/splinting, local wound care and antibiotic therapy. The patient underwent a double local random rhomboid and monolobe flap closures (*B*) with percutaneous tendo-Achilles lengthening and application of a circular external fixation device for surgical offloading (*C–F*). Note that medial and lateral struts (*D, E*) placement that allow for continuous correction of the tendo-Achilles lengthening and alignment of the foot in the desired anatomic position and the struts that are used for surgical offloading (*F*) elevating the heel from any contact surfaces by preventing a weight-bearing status and allowing for direct visualization of the flap and access to local wound care if needed.

decreases the wound sizes more effectively as compared with traditional, nonsurgical offloading. It is especially useful in cases of severely infected and complicated wounds that require continuous monitoring and direct access to the wound site for care. External fixation also has been shown to increase the survival rate of lower extremity flaps by providing direct visualization of the flap for continuous assessment and to prevent direct pressure on the flap[1,6,7] (**Fig. 3**).

External fixation is relatively contraindicated in patients who cannot tolerate the procedure, patients at risk for nonadherence to the treatment and rigorous postoperative course, individuals with untreated peripheral vascular disease, a nonsalvageable limb, or the presence of internal hardware that prohibits proper wire or pin placement. Patient selection and preoperative planning are crucial before application of external fixation to optimize the success rate of diabetic limb salvage and prevent the need for an amputation. External fixation application in diabetic foot ulcerations has promising results with positive outcomes in diabetic limb preservation.[8,9]

SUMMARY

External fixation has become extremely useful in the management of complicated diabetic foot wounds and has contributed greatly to limb preservation through its advantages in offloading and deformity correction. Although there is a risk of complications associated with this procedure, these may be avoided through appropriate surgical training, careful patient selection, and thorough perioperative care.

REFERENCES

1. Nayak B, Mahapatra KC. Das Management of complex diabetic foot wound by external fixation: an effective way for limb salvage. J Health Specialties 2016; 4(2):128.
2. Patro B, Surana P, Mahapatra KC. A study of the efficacy of external fixation in healing large, deep and unstable diabetic foot wounds. Int Surg J 2019;6(3): 669–74.
3. Ramanujam C, Facaros Z, Zgonis T. External fixation for surgical offloading of diabetic soft tissue reconstruction. Clin Podiatr Med Surg 2011 Jan;28(1):211–6.
4. Clark J, Mills J, Armstrong D. A method of external fixation to offload and protect the foot following reconstruction in high-risk patients: the SALSA stand. Eplasty 2009;9:e21.
5. Clemens MW, Parikh P, Hall MM, et al. External fixators as an adjunct to wound healing. Foot Ankle Clin 2008;13:145–56.
6. Kachare Swapnil D, Vivace Bradley J, Henderson Joshua T, et al. Kickstand external fixator for immobilization following free flap plantar Calcaneal reconstruction. Eplasty 2019;19:e11.
7. Oznur A, Zgonis T. Closure of major diabetic foot wounds with external fixation. Clin Podiatr Med Surg 2007;24(3):519–928.
8. Lowenberg DW, Sadeghi C, Brooks D, et al. Use of circular external fixation to maintain foot position during free tissue transfer to the foot and ankle. Microsurgery 2008;28:623–7.
9. Zgonis T, Oznur A, Roukis TS. A novel technique for closing difficult diabetic cleft foot wounds with skin grafting and a ring-type external fixation system. Oper Tech Orthop 2006;16:38–43.

Printed and bound by CPI Group (UK) Ltd, Croydon, CR0 4YY

03/10/2024

01040406-0002